Physical
Therapy for
the Cancer
Patient

CLINICS IN PHYSICAL THERAPY

26-50

Forthcoming Volumes in the Series

Physical Therapy for the Cancer Patient

Edited by

Charles L. McGarvey III, M.S., P.T.

Chief, Physical Therapy Section
Department of Rehabilitation Medicine
Warren G. Magnuson Clinical Center
National Institutes of Health
Bethesda, Maryland
Clinical Associate Professor of Physical Therapy
Sargent College of Allied Health Professions
Boston University
Boston, Massachusetts
Past President
Oncology Section
American Physical Therapy Association Inc.
Alexandria, Virginia

CHURCHILL LIVINGSTONE

NEW YORK, EDINBURGH, LONDON, MELBOURNE

Library of Congress Cataloging-in-Publication Data

Physical therapy for the cancer patient / edited by Charles L.
   McGarvey III.
    p.   cm.—(Clinics in physical therapy)
   Includes bibliographical references.
   ISBN 0-443-08667-2
   1. Cancer—Physical therapy.   2. Cancer—Patients—Rehabilitation.
I. McGarvey, Charles L.   II. Series.
   [DNLM: 1. Neoplasms—rehabilitation.   2. Physical Therapy.   W1
CL831CN / QZ 266 P5782]
RC271.P44P48   1990
616.99'4062—dc20
DNLM/DLC
for Library of Congress   90-32270
                                                                          CIP

© **Churchill Livingstone Inc. 1990**

This book was edited in the editor's private capacity. No official support or
endorsement by the United States Department of Health and Human Services is
intended or should be inferred. The information presented in this text reflects the
views of the authors and not necessarily those of the National Institutes of Health
or the United States Public Health Service.

Distributed in the United Kingdom by Churchill Livingstone, Robert Stevenson
House, 1–3 Baxter's Place, Leith Walk, Edinburgh EH1 3AF, and by associated
companies, branches, and representatives throughout the world.

Accurate indications, adverse reactions, and dosage schedules for drugs are
provided in this book, but it is possible that they may change. The reader is urged
to review the package information data of the manufacturers of the medications
mentioned.

The Publishers have made every effort to trace the copyright holders for borrowed
material. If they have inadvertently overlooked any, they will be pleased to make
the necessary arrangements at the first opportunity.

Acquisitions Editor: *Kim Loretucci*
Copy Editor: *Elizabeth Bowman*
Production Designer: *Angela Cirnigliaro*
Production Supervisor: *Jeanine Furino*

Printed in the United States of America

First published in 1990

To Trudy and Megan

May the time spent away from you
to prepare this book be worthy
of its intended purpose

Contributors

Joyce L. Adcock, M.A., P.T.
Director, Physical Therapy, Jenkintown Rehabilitation Services, Jenkintown, Pennsylvania

Kathleen Chesney, P.T.
City of Hope National Medical Center, Duarte, California

Cheryl Gahagen, M.S., P.T.
Senior Physical Therapist, City of Hope National Medical Center, Duarte, California

Carolyn Cook Gotay, Ph.D.
Visiting Scholar, Office of Research Evaluation and Computer Resources, University of California, San Francisco, School of Nursing, San Francisco, California

Lauren Holtzman, M.A., P.T.
Currently in private practice; formerly Senior Physical Therapist, Oncology Service, Department of Rehabilitation Medicine, Johns Hopkins Hospital, Baltimore, Maryland

Marsha H. Lampert, P.T.
Clinical Coordinator, Physical Therapy Service, Department of Rehabilitation Medicine, National Institutes of Health, Bethesda, Maryland

Sharon Last, P.T.
President, Oakland Rehabilitation Systems, P.C., Southfield, Michigan

Charles L. McGarvey III, M.S., P.T.
Chief, Physical Therapy Section, Department of Rehabilitation Medicine, Warren G. Magnuson Clinical Center, National Institutes of Health, Bethesda, Maryland; Clinical Associate Professor of Physical Therapy, Sargent College of Allied Health Professions, Boston University, Boston, Massachusetts; Past President, Oncology Section, American Physical Therapy Association Inc., Alexandria, Virginia

Rick Reuss, P.T.
Director, Department of Physical Therapy, The King's Daughters' Hospital, Madison, Indiana

William Lee Roberts, M.P.T.
Director, Rehabilitative Services, H. Lee Moffitt Cancer Center and Research Institute, Tampa, Florida

Julia H. Rowland, Ph.D.
Clinical Assistant Attending Psychologist, Psychiatry Service, Department of Neurology, Memorial Sloan-Kettering Cancer Center; Instructor of Psychology in Psychiatry, Department of Psychiatry, Cornell University Medical College, New York, New York

Bernadette D. Shea, P.T.
Administrative Coordinator and Chief Physical Therapist, Rehabilitation Service, Memorial Sloan-Kettering Cancer Center, New York, New York

Georgann Vlad, M.A., P.T.
Department of Physical Therapy, University of Southern California, Los Angeles, California

Jeri F. Walton, P.T.
Founder and Past President, Oncology Section, American Physical Therapy Association Inc., Alexandria, Virginia

Preface

Cancer remains the second leading cause of mortality in the United States. Historically, cancer research has concentrated on its cause, detection, and medical treatment. While progress has been made in the identification of carcinogens, much more progress has been achieved in early detection and medical treatments as a result of advances in biologic and biomedical engineering. These technical improvements have resulted in increased survival rates for a number of cancer patients. Current statistics reflect that over 5 million Americans are alive today with a diagnosis of cancer, 3 million with a history of 5 years or more. Cancer is generally a disease affecting the elderly, and current projections are that one fifth of the U.S. population will be 65 or older by the year 2040.

In light of these trends, physical therapists will be called upon to play a more active role in the acute and chronic care of these cancer survivors. Administration of proper therapeutic modalities requires a working knowledge of the disease, its medical management, and specific effects of antineoplastic procedures. Establishment of short- and long-term goals for these patients requires a focus on functional issues related to the quality of remaining life, whether it be six months or six years. Educationally, physical therapy programs may need to include additional courses, or possibly an area of specialization, in oncology. Unfortunately there are very few published studies investigating physical therapy and oncology to support future reimbursement issues. Studies related to lost hours of work, effects of exercise, and pain control for cancer patients are sorely needed. Currently less than 1 percent of all research monies budgeted by the National Cancer Institute involve investigation in areas of cancer rehabilitation.

The intention of this text is to provide the physical therapist and physical therapy assistant or student with a general appreciation of oncology and how it relates to the profession of physical therapy. Following an introduction to basic oncology principles and therapeutic procedures, clinical chapters describe current rehabilitation concepts involved in the assessment and treatment of various types of cancer patients. The final chapters discuss psychosocial issues and factors related to the care of the terminally ill patient in the hospice or at home.

This text will serve as one of the few clinical reference sources that addresses the needs of the cancer patient from a physical therapy perspective.

Special thanks to Kim Loretucci, Carol Bader, and the Churchill Livingstone staff for the assistance provided in the production of this volume.

Charles L. McGarvey III, M.S., P.T.

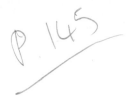

Contents

1 | Oncology: Principles and Management

Charles L. McGarvey III
Jeri F. Walton

GENERAL STATISTICS

Cancer statistics have been collected by the federal government since 1950. From 1950 through 1973 the National Cancer Institute (NCI) monitored various statistics related to incidence and mortality rates of cancer in the United States using data compiled from selected cities and states. This information was useful in establishing baseline data for the prevalence of this disease process in the United States but was limited in the degree of sophistication necessary to justify development of major research or treatment intervention.

Beginning in 1973, the NCI has presented data compiled through the Surveillance, Epidemiology, and End Results (SEER) program. These data, as prepared by the NCI's Division of Cancer Prevention and Control and the Division of Cancer Treatment, reflect the incidence of cancer from 11 population-based registries, age-adjusted to the 1970 census, and represent roughly 10 percent of the U.S. population.

The traditional source of mortality statistics has been a sister agency, the National Center for Health Statistics (NCHS). These data are based on death certificates and are also age-adjusted to the 1970 census.

This chapter was written in the author's private capacity. No official support or endorsement by the United States Department of Health and Human Services is intended or should be inferred. The information presented in this chapter reflects the views of the authors and not necessarily those of the National Institutes of Health or the United States Public Health Service.

A comprehensive report detailing cancer trends, incidence, mortality, and survival is produced each year by NCI and published each spring under the title Annual Cancer Statistics Review.[1,2] It is from these data that the American Cancer Society (ACS) extrapolates information for the estimates of incidence and mortality that it publishes annually in Cancer Facts and Figures.[3] This publication has become the most frequently cited source for statistical data related to the prevalence and impact of cancer. One should appreciate that while these data are regarded as estimates, they do represent an accurate sampling of the American population and have been carefully collated and analyzed since 1976.

The following statistics are those reported in 1989 in Cancer Facts and Figures. It should be noted that these figures do not reflect new cases of nonmelanoma skin cancer or carcinoma in situ, which account for an estimated 500,000 new cases annually.

Incidence

Of Americans alive today, 76 million, representing roughly one-third of our current population, will develop cancer in their lifetime, and cancer will strike three out of four families. In 1989 it was projected that just over 1 million (1,010,000) new cases of cancer would be diagnosed. This figure has consistently increased by approximately 25,000 each year since 1986.

Mortality

It has been estimated that in 1990 cancer, regarded as the second highest killer of Americans, will kill 510,000 persons in the United States—one person every 62 seconds. While statistics related to incidence and mortality remain vital, statistics related to cure and length of survival have become increasingly important to rehabilitation personnel assessing the potential of these patients to resume or adapt their lifestyles following diagnosis and treatment.

Cure, as defined by the ACS, occurs in "a patient with no evidence of disease and having the same life expectancy as a person who never had cancer." The term may be further defined for most forms of cancer as 5 years without symptoms. Qualifications to this time requirement include exceptions based on the type of cancer diagnosed. Investigators involved in clinical research trials will often use the terms *partial remission* or *complete remission* as indicators of survival or cure as related to time.

Regarding survival, there are over 5 million Americans alive today with a history of cancer and 3 million with a diagnosis made at least 5 years ago. The trend in survival has gradually increased every year since 1960 to a 4 in 10, or 40 percent, *observed survival rate.* When adjusted to normal life expectancy (to allow for cancer patients who die of other causes such as heart disease or accidents), this figure climbs to 49 percent and is termed *relative survival rate*

(Fig. 1-1). These increases in survival rates are attributed to a host of factors, including earlier detection through improved medical screening and diagnostic technology, improvement in medical management (surgery, radiation, chemotherapy) and education.

These statistics indicate that while incidence and mortality of all cancer cases continue to increase, rates of patient survival for 5 or more years are also increasing. Combined with the fact that more Americans are living longer, the question of quality of remaining life is fast becoming the focus of many health care disciplines. A general description of the more common musculoskeletal deficits and the rehabilitation intervention have been previously presented by Gerber and McGarvey.[4]

Politically, Congress has been struggling with the concept of a fully funded catastrophic health care plan and its potential impact on the nation's economy. Economically, insurance carriers are reexamining their policies and liabilities related to reimbursement of cancer-related health care costs.

Recent impact of the federal Diagnosis Related Group (DRG) regulations on hospital admission and discharge rates, combined with the increasing geriatric population, is creating an increased need for home health care services. Information reported by the NCHS indicates overall medical costs for cancer at $71.6 billion in 1985. $21.8 billion for direct costs, $8.6 billion for so called morbidity costs (cost of lost productivity) and $41.2 billion for mortality costs. Cancer accounts for roughly 10 percent of the total cost of all diseases in the United States. These factors and many others will require allied health care professionals to be well educated in the medical management and expected rehabilitation goals of cancer patients.

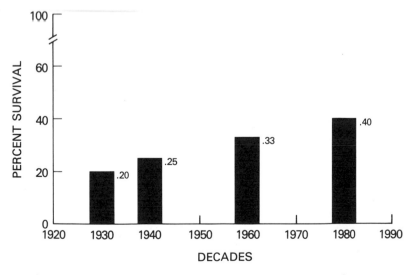

Fig. 1-1. Relative survival trends. (From American Cancer Society,[3] with permission.)

PRINCIPLES OF CELLULAR AND TISSUE CHANGE

To understand the patient with cancer one must understand the pathology of cancer.[5]

Cancer is a very complex group of diseases that is difficult to define; indeed, there is no single definition that is universally accepted. It consists of over 250 types of neoplasms characterized by the uncontrolled spread of abnormal cells, which invade and destroy normal tissue. Left untreated, it can result in the death of the host organism.[6,7] Cancer is a disease of the cell in which the normal mechanisms of control of growth and proliferation are disturbed, which results in distinctive morphologic alterations of the cell and aberrations of tissue patterns. The diagnosis of cancer, as well as many of its medical treatments, is based upon these cytologic and histologic alterations.[6] It is only through an understanding of the basic principles of cellular and tissue changes that one can begin to understand the natural history of the disease, the principles upon which its treatment is based, and the possible outcomes for the patient. This knowledge is of significant importance to rehabilitation professionals, as they assist patients to realistically identify and achieve goals within their abilities and prognoses.

Cell Growth

All mammalian cells have the capacity to divide and enter the cell cycle. *The cell cycle* is defined by Baserga[8] as "the interval between the midpoint of mitosis and the midpoint of the subsequent mitosis in one daughter cell or both." However, an understanding of the cell cycle requires knowledge of the cellular and biochemical aspects that regulate cell growth, whether that growth is normal or abnormal.[8] This knowledge is vital to an understanding of the disease of cancer and its principles of treatment. The cell cycle is usually represented by a circle (Fig. 1-2) and divided into four stages, G1, S (DNA synthesis), G2, and M (mitosis). G1 is the "gap" between division and S and G2 is that between S and M.[9]

All tissue populations (normal and abnormal) consist of a mixture of three different cell populations (Fig. 1-3). *Continuously dividing cells* are those that advance from one mitosis to the next within a short time. These are the cells that supply new cells for growing tissue, for tissue repair, or following normal cell

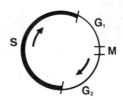

Fig. 1-2.   The cell cycle.

death. These dividing cells are found in tissues as stem cells or as cells that are in a partially differentiated compartment. Rapidly proliferating bone marrow cells are an example of continuously dividing cells. *Cells that differentiate* leave the cell cycle after a certain number of divisions and differentiate into specific tissue types. These cells are destined to die without dividing again and have specific functions in the tissue that assist in maintaining the normal life of the host. An example of a differentiated type of cell is the granulocyte, a nondividing mature cell in the bone marrow. *G0, or dormant, cells* leave the cell cycle temporarily and remain dormant until environmental conditions stimulate their reentry into the cycle. The stem cells in the bone marrow are an example.[8]

As stated previously, these three cell populations are present in varying proportions in every tissue. In normal cell division, the majority of cells progress, from G1 to differentiation into a specific cell type and eventually to death. Cancer cells, however, do not differentiate but remain in a continuous phase of cell division. This is termed *anaplasia* and is a hallmark of malignancy and one of the criteria used by the pathologist for diagnosis. Cancer cells also lose other normal cell characteristics, as discussed below.

Tissue Growth

Tissues grow primarily through an increase in the number of cells. In normal tissues this occurs during embryogenesis, childhood, liver regeneration, etc. In cancer the normal cell growth controls have been disrupted, resulting in an imbalance in the tissue growth control mechanisms and an increase in the *total* number of cells.

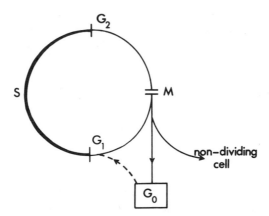

Fig. 1-3. Cell populations and the phases of the cell cycle. Continuously dividing cells go around the cell cycle from one mitosis (M) to the next. Nondividing cells have left the cycle and are destined to die without dividing again. Quiescent G_0 cells are neither cycling nor dying and can be induced to reenter the cycle by an appropriate stimulus. (From Baserga,[8] with permission.)

Normal and abnormal tissue growth both depend on three cell population functions: the cell cycle time, the growth fraction, and the rate of cell loss. The *cell cycle time* is the interval between mitoses in cycling cells. The shorter the interval, the faster the cells are produced. The *growth fraction* is the fraction of the total cell population that is cycling cells. The larger the fraction, the faster the increase in cell number. The *rate of cell loss* is the fraction of cells that die or migrate to other tissues.[8,10]

In an adult there is no growth, and the number of cells produced per unit of time is equal to the number that die. Normal tissues and organs are in a steady state. Cancer cells are *not* in a steady state, but instead cell growth continues uncontrolled. The amount of cell growth is determined by the rate of cell growth minus that of cell loss.[8]

HISTOLOGIC AND CYTOLOGIC FEATURES OF MALIGNANCY

Malignant tumors vary considerably in morphology but certain features are commonly found. As Kempson and Hendrickson have stated, "No single architectural or cytologic feature is diagnostic of malignancy."[11] Many tumors will demonstrate most malignant criteria, but some will have only a few, and some benign tumors will display some of the morphologic features of cancer.

The principal histologic and cytologic features of malignancy include the following:

1. *Uncontrolled cellular proliferation*. Cancer cells divide relentlessly and do not differentiate. They have a high mitotic rate (i.e., a large proportion of the cells are undergoing mitosis at any one time). Cancer cells also lack contact inhibition (i.e., they do not have the normal control mechanisms that inhibit continued cell growth when cell membrane contact is made with other cells). The cells instead begin to pile up on each other.

2. *Invasiveness*. Cancer cells move through basement membranes and infiltrate and destroy surrounding tissue, often including vascular and lymphatic channels. This allows, for example, a tumor composed of breast tissue to move into the adjacent muscle, resulting in destruction of that tissue.

3. *Destruction of normal tissue*. Cancer cells destroy normal tissue as a result of their infiltrative and invasive characteristics. Tissue destruction may be secondary to the release of lytic substances by the tumor, pressure from the buildup of cells, competition for nutrients, or combinations of these and other effects.[12]

4. *Atypical tissue structure (anaplasia)*. Anaplasia is a change in normal cell growth patterns whereby basal generative cells fail to differentiate into functional cells. Cancer cells often display marked anaplasia. Anaplasia is considered a hallmark of malignancy when seen in biopsied tissue.[13]

5. *Pleomorphism*. Cancer cells often display a variety of cell shapes. Cellular patterns may vary from area to area in the same tumor, and individual tumors may vary considerably in their appearance.

6. *Aneuploidy*. Malignant cells demonstrate abnormal DNA content and may have multiple nucleoli within cell nuclei and abnormal mitotic figures.

7. *Metastases*. Cancer cells are poorly adherent, readily detached, and highly mobile. They are able to move from the tissue of origin, usually along the path of least resistance (through lymphatic or vascular channels), to other tissues. They may lie dormant in the other tissues or may begin to multiply and invade that tissue. It is important to remember that the tissue type of the tumor is always the tissue of origin even though it may have metastasized into other tissues.

CLINICAL DIAGNOSIS OF CANCER

At present the diagnosis of cancer must be made histologically; that is, the cancerous cells must be observed under the microscope. Generally speaking, a tumor can be diagnosed clinically when approximately 1×10^9 (1 billion) cells at one site produce a mass about 1 cm in diameter. Unfortunately, many patients do not seek medical attention until the tumor is considerably larger than 1×10^9 cells.[14] The goal in the medical treatment of cancer is to destroy enough of the malignant cells to decrease the tumor burden to a level at which the patient's own immune system can destroy any remaining abnormal cells. When fewer than 1×10^9 cancer cells are present in the patient and the clinician is unable to find any evidence of disease, the patient is said to be in *clinical remission* or to have *no evidence of disease*. A patient in clinical remission may have microscopic disease that is not detectable by any current diagnostic method.

THE ROLE OF THE IMMUNE SYSTEM

The immune system is thought to play a very important but not well understood role in the development of cancer in a host. It is generally accepted that at any one time everyone has cells that have lost their normal control mechanisms and have the characteristics of cancer cells. In a healthy person these abnormal cells are identified by the highly complex immune system and are destroyed.[10,15] For unknown reasons, in certain individuals these abnormal cells proliferate until they are too numerous for the immune system to destroy.[7,15] It is well documented that those persons who are immunosuppressed, congenitally or therapeutically, are at much higher risk for developing cancer.[10,13,15-18] Stress may also decrease the immune response and create an environment more favorable to the development of cancer. Cancer incidence is higher in the very young and very old (i.e., at those ages at which the immune system is not as efficient as during the middle years of life). The development of immunotherapy as a medical treatment for cancer patients is based on the hope of enhancing the patient's own immune system to the point that it can then recognize and destroy any and all cancer cells.

CLASSIFICATION OF TUMORS

The large variety of tumors has necessitated a method of classification to assist those working in oncology with discussions and comparisons of different tumors and their responses. Classification of neoplasms has become a very important aspect of oncologic research and patient care. It attempts to ensure, for both clinical and research purposes, that comparisons are made between tumors of similar type and characteristics. Many different methods of classification have been developed over the years and have become increasingly complex as scientists learn more and more about specific tumor types.

The objectives of classification are to (1) aid the clinician in planning treatment; (2) give an indication of prognosis; (3) assist in the evaluation of treatment results; (4) facilitate exchange of information between treatment centers and professionals; and (5) assist in the continuing investigation of cancer.[19,20] In brief, accurate classification benefits all who are involved by ensuring they are comparing "apples with apples" when discussing different types of cancers and their respective responses to treatment.

Current classification is based upon

1.   Histogenesis: tissue of origin and cell type
2.   Biologic behavior: benign or malignant
3.   Anatomic site: staging
4.   Degree of differentiation[6]

Histogenesis

Tumors can arise from virtually all types of normal tissue and usually retain enough features of the normal cell and tissue patterns to resemble their tissue of origin.[6] However, since some tumors may be highly anaplastic and consist of primitive germlike cells, it is at times difficult to determine the specific tissue of origin; hence the term *tumor of unknown origin.*

Benign tumors are usually named by adding the suffix *-oma* to the name of a cell or tissue type (e.g., lip*oma,* neur*oma*). Malignant tumors are divided into sarcomas, those of mesenchymal origin, and carcinomas, those that arise from epithelial tissue. These terms are then used with the tissue or cell of origin (e.g., adenocarcinoma, osteosarcoma). There are many exceptions to this, however, exampified by those tumors of hematopoietic and lymphocytic origin that are classified separately and by those tumors with specific eponyms (e.g., Hodgkin's disease and Ewing's sarcoma).[6]

Biologic Behavior

The biologic behavior of the tumor cells determines whether the tumor is benign or malignant. Benign tumors are generally innocuous and harmless to the host, while malignant tumors are agressive neoplasms, which if left untreated generally result in metastases and death.[6]

Anatomic Staging

Anatomic staging attempts to quantify the extent of disease in the patient. It provides a rough estimate of the number of cancer cells present and helps to determine the approximate prognosis and the most appropriate methods of treatment. Initial staging is always done at the time of diagnosis but may be revised following further studies or progression of the patient's disease. Staging is limited by the medical technology available and the judgment of the physician in determining how much information is needed to serve the best interest of the patient without subjecting the patient to unnecessary procedures and expense. Staging is a vital step in the treatment of the cancer patient, as it is one of the fundamental bases for determining prognosis and medical management.

Historically, cancer staging was described by the numerals *I* through *IV*, which are often still used clinically. These traditional stages are as follows:

Stage I: Cancer is limited to the organ in which it develops.

Stage II: The tumor is spread beyond the primary site but remains in the same anatomic region. There is some local invasion of the organ or the immediately adjacent areas. There may be first-stage lymph node spread with microinvasion of the lymphatics.

Stage III: The tumor has spread to the region surrounding the primary organ. There is a high probability of microscopic metastatic disease.

Stage IV: Metastatic disease is present beyond the local site. Cancer cells are present throughout the entire organism, and there is little chance for cure.

Recently the staging process has become much more sophisticated and now provides clinicians and researchers with more specific comparisons of tumors and responses to treatment methods. Today, additional criteria used include the extent of the primary tumor (T), the absence or presence and extent of regional lymph node metastases (N), and the presence or absence of distant metastases (M).[20] This method, termed the *TNM* classification, is now in widespread clinical use and is accepted as the required classification in many situations for admitting patients into clinical research treatment protocols.

TNM staging is currently the acceptable method of staging. It was developed over a number of years by various organizations, and a consensus of criteria was defined in 1988 by the American Joint Committee on Cancer (AJCC).[20] This staging classification is "based on the premise that cancers of similar histology or site of origin share similar patterns of growth and extension. The size of the untreated primary cancer or tumor (T) increases progressively, and at some point in time regional lymph node involvement (N) and, finally, distant metastases (M) occur"[20] (Fig. 1-4). Exact specifications are defined for each cancer type, and one must refer to the AJCC Manual for Staging of Cancer[20] for those definitions.

T defines the primary tumor by depth of invasion, surface spread, and size and is expressed as T1, T2, T3, or T4; T1 denotes a small tumor and T4 the most extensive. Exact criteria exist for each definition, which varies with the specific organ site. N defines the extent of nodal disease and is expressed as N0, N1, N2,

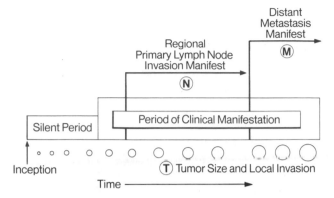

Fig. 1-4. The evolution of the TNM stages of cancer. (From Beahrs et al.,[20] with permission.)

or N3; N0 indicates no evidence of disease and N3 indicates multiple fixed nodes usually greater than 5 cm. Once again the definition varies with each specific organ site. M is expressed as either M0 or M+, meaning simply the absence or presence, respectively, of metastasis.[21]

Clinically, TNM classifications may be combined with the traditional groupings. The following examples help to explain this concept and define the characteristics of possible stage groupings[20]:

1. *Stage I, T1, N0, M0:* Clinical examination reveals a mass limited to organ of origin. The lesion is operable and resectable with only local involvement, and there is no nodal or vascular spread. This stage affords the best chance for survival (70 to 90 percent).

2. *Stage II, T2, N1, M0:* Clinical examination shows evidence of local spread into surrounding tissue and first station lymph nodes. The lesion is operable and resectable, but because of greater local extent there is uncertainty about completeness of removal. The specimen shows evidence of microinvasion into capsule and lymphatics. This stage affords a good chance of survival (about 50 ± 5 percent).

3. *Stage III, T3, N2, M0:* Clinical examination reveals an extensive primary tumor with fixation to deeper structures, bone invasion, and lymph nodes of similar nature. The lesion is operable but not resectable, and gross disease is left behind. This stage affords some chance of survival (20 ± 5 percent).

4. *Stage IV, T4, N3, M+:* Evidence of distant metastases beyond the local site or organ. The primary lesion is inoperable. There is little to no chance for survival in most cases (<5 percent).

Degree of Differentiation

Determination of the degree of differentiation of the cancer cells is an aspect of tumor classification that is of major importance in determining the patient's prognosis. It is an expression of the histopathology of the tumor and helps to define its degree of malignancy. It is used in various tumor types, particularly those of the testes, ovaries, and brain. The degree of differentiation is the *grade* of the tumor. Since the more anaplastic the cells, the more malignant the tumor, the grade is also an expression of the tumor's degree of malignancy.

The grade is expressed either numerically, as I, II, III, or IV, or descriptively, as well, moderately, or poorly differentiated. Tumors of numerical grades I and II, or well differentiated, are those that cytologically and histologically deviate least from normal. Tumors of grades III and IV, or poorly differentiated, are the most anaplastic and bear the least resemblance to normal cellular and tissue patterns. In general, the lower the grade, the better the prognosis, and the higher the grade, the poorer the prognosis.[2]

It is important to point out that since cells undergoing mitosis are usually more sensitive to radiation therapy and chemotherapy, tumors that are more anaplastic sometimes respond better to these treatments. This fact has been used very effectively in the treatment of some highly malignant tumors that would otherwise have a very poor prognosis.

ANTINEOPLASTIC STRATEGIES

The treatment of cancer is determined by various factors, including the type and location of the primary tumor and the stage and grade of disease. Other factors, such as the patient's general health and age and the patient's and family's beliefs and desires, also play a major role.

The four methods of treatment for cancer are surgery, chemotherapy, radiation therapy, and immunotherapy. Surgery has the goal of excising as many of the cancerous cells as possible, often as a means of cure but also as a method of debulking the tumor prior to radiation, chemotherapy, or immunotherapy. Radiation therapy uses ionizing radiation to destroy tumor cells, sparing most normal cells, and affects only those tissues directly exposed to the treatment beam. Chemotherapy uses toxic chemicals systemically to kill macro- or microscopic cancer cells. Immunotherapy is currently largely experimental, but some believe it to hold the most promise for curative breakthroughs. It is based on the assumption that the patient's own immune system can be enhanced to kill any remaining cancer cells.

Although rehabilitation professionals are not primarily involved in the curative aspects of cancer treatment, it is very important that they know and understand the medical basis of oncology. They need to be able to understand what the patient is experiencing and has experienced and what effect medical treatments and tests might have on the patient's response to the rehabilitation process.

Medical information that affects the rehabilitation process includes:

1. *Primary diagnosis:* What organ and cell type was originally affected? What is the natural history of cancer of that organ and cell type?

2. *Stage of disease:* How far advanced was the original tumor? What tissues and organs were involved?

3. *Type of surgery:* What tissue structures were excised, resected, etc.? Did the surgery include a lymphadenectomy?

4. *Radiation therapy:* What were the fields (i.e., what tissues were involved)? What are the possible side effects?

5. *Chemotherapy:* What agents were used? What are the possible short- and long-term side effects?

6. *Blood counts:* What are the patient's blood counts, including red blood cells, hematocrit, white blood cells, and platelets?

7. *Radiographic results:* What are the findings of x-ray examination and those of other diagnostic radiographic tests? Are there metastases in bones or other areas affecting the patient's physical abilities?

8. *Prognosis:* What is the patient's short- and long-term prognosis? What are the most important functional goals?

This information can assist rehabilitation professionals to properly assess the patient's functional abilities and needs and to establish an effective, realistic, achievable rehabilitation program. It is extremely important that the rehabilitation professionals play an active role in the care of the cancer patient, and only with a good understanding of the disease and its treatment is this possible.

Surgery

In an overview of surgical oncology, the prominent oncologists McKenna and McKenna state that surgery, "cures twice as many patients as all modalities (i.e., radiotherapy and chemotherapy) combined."[22] This traditional view of the role of the surgeon in the primary management of cancers is generally supported by others.[23-25] Recently, however, data from carefully controlled clinical trials have led McKenna and others to recognize the potential value of adjuvant therapies, primarily in the control of micrometastatic disease but also as a viable option prior to a surgical procedure. In the following statement the McKennas appear to summarize the current philosophy of some surgical oncologists:

> The role of the surgeon in the treatment of cancer is at a crossroad. During the era of single modality treatment surgery assumed the dominant role, since its results were clearly superior to chemotherapy and radiotherapy. Despite the successful control of local and regional disease by surgery, patients often subsequently died of metastatic disease. It is now well recognized that many cases of cancer are disseminated at the time of diagnosis even though the metastases are subclinical and undetectable. Systemic treatment is necessary to cure such patients, so we are now entering the era of multimodality treatment for cancer. The surgeon is now faced with the choice of assuming a secondary role in cancer treatment or

expanding his role in cancer treatment by continuing to perform curative operations in appropriate patients and developing creative new roles for surgery to cure or palliate cancer patients in coordination with the efforts of a multidisciplinary team.[22]

In addition, McKenna states

The surgeon who becomes an active member of the cancer team will have an expanded role in the total care of the patient. He will use a combination of "radical" and "conservative" procedures within the context of this multidisciplinary treatment. With longer survival for cancer patients, many new situations arise in which surgical intervention might be appropriate for rejecting metastasis, restaging, debulking and treating a variety of oncologic emergencies.[22]

Surgical intervention can be divided into four basic areas: diagnosis, clinical staging, treatment, and reconstruction.

Diagnosis

In the diagnostic phase, the surgeon plays an important role in the investigation of a neoplasm by providing the pathologist with a sample of the tumor. Diagnosis of the tumor is confirmed histologically by an experienced pathologist. Sampling of the tumor is accomplished through biopsy. The following are examples of biopsy techniques used by surgeons to obtain sufficient tumor tissue to enable the pathologist to make an accurate diagnosis.

1. Cytologic procedures
    a) Direct smear
    b) Fluid aspiration
    c) Aspiration needle biopsy
    d) Cutting needle biopsy
    e) Endoscopic biopsy
2. Open biopsy procedures
    a) Incisional biopsy
    b) Excisional biopsy

The decision of which biopsy procedure to employ is not simple and may even require a major surgical process. The surgeon must weigh the advantages versus the disadvantages of each technique, as the possibility of contamination of surrounding tissue or insufficient retrieval of specimen necessary for diagnosis may significantly affect treatment choice and final outcome. A thorough explanation of each biopsy procedure and its relative merit is contained in most comprehensive surgical oncology textbooks.[23,26,27]

Clinical Staging

The second phase of surgical intervention involves clinical staging, the process by which all known information regarding the patient and the neoplasm is presented in order to determine the type, extent, and aggressiveness of the tumor. On the basis of this information, the most definitive strategy necessary to achieve total ablation of the disease within the greatest allowable risk to the patient is decided. Opinions as to whether there are realistic choices for cure versus palliation may be offered by practitioners of the various disciplines at this time. Again, the decision is not an easy one; while medical technology has advanced rapidly over the years, it has not totally replaced the eyes, hands, or experience of a skilled surgeon in making the final decision as to whether a tumor is indeed resectable or whether there is evidence of gross metastatic disease in surrounding tissue that was previously undetected by machine or laboratory test.

Treatment

The third surgical phase involves definitive treatment. Historically, surgical treatment for the cure of primary cancers had been the accepted and most practiced strategy. Palliative surgery had also been practiced to allow patients as much comfort as possible during their remaining life. More recently, controversy regarding the most appropriate type of surgery for treatment of specific cancers has surfaced.[28] Procedures for the aggressive treatment of metastatic disease have also been advocated.[29]

In general, surgical procedures requiring resection of a low-grade tumor with a small margin of "normal tissue" and not involving surrounding organs are referred to as *local excisions*. Modifications of this procedure, involving removal of additional tissue, as in surgery of sarcomas, have led to the adoption of the term *wide local excision*. These procedures are sometimes also classified as excisional biopsy technique.

High-grade malignancies and those in close proximity to regional nodes may require an *en bloc* or block dissection. In this procedure the tumor, organ of origin, and regional nodes may be resected as a whole specimen. En bloc dissections may necessitate the removal of muscle, nerve, bone, or lymphatics as a single unit, resulting in the amputation or gross functional disability of the residual limb.

Additional Surgical Procedures. Other surgical techniques, including electrosurgery, cryosurgery, chemosurgery, laser surgery, isolation perfusion, intra-arterial infusion, and debulking, have been used extensively over the past 20 years in one form or another for various benign and malignant neoplasms. The main objective of such procedures is to spare as much "normal" tissue as possible. The safety and efficacy of each is dependent on tumor type, proximity to other vital organs, and relative skill of the surgeon.

Reconstruction

The fourth and final phase, reconstructive surgery, may or may not be performed. As a result of improvements in surgical technique and in response to patients' requests, surgeons have developed increasing expertise in the cosmetic reconstruction of organ systems and extremities. Classic examples of reconstruction surgery include augmentation mammoplasty utilizing silicone implants, muscle flap transfers, or subcutaneous soft tissue expansion. Other examples include reconstruction of head and neck compartments and limb-sparing procedures. The latter operations employ the same general techniques practiced in joint replacement surgery as they involve implantation of a prosthetic component to substitute for the joint that was resected. The objective of these procedures is to provide the patient with the best aesthetic and functional result possible without sacrificing the intent of the primary surgery. Cosmesis, a component of quality of life, has become an extremely important factor to those cancer patients surviving primary treatment of their disease.

Chemotherapy

The term *chemotherapy* is defined in the 27th edition of Dorland's Medical Dictionary as "the treatment of disease by chemical agents; first applied to use of chemicals that affect the causative organism unfavorably but do not harm the patient." While it is correct that cancer is treated by chemical agents, the claim that these chemicals do not harm the patient is easily challenged.

Since the early 1940s cancer chemotherapy has become a science dedicated to understanding the biology of normal cells and their interaction with specific chemical toxins in relation to the management of cancer. Often classified as adjuvant therapy, chemotherapy has become one of the major strategies employed in the management of neoplastic disease.

Systemic cytotoxic chemicals have been developed and used predominantly to treat disseminated metastatic disease. Recently, however, efforts have been made to use these drugs preoperatively in an attempt to reduce tumor size and thus facilitate easier surgical resection and promote earlier control of metastatic spread. Moreover in cases involving lymphomas and leukemias, chemotherapy is recognized as the primary treatment choice.

Currently over 50 nonhormonal cytotoxic agents with demonstrated antitumor activity are available.[30] They are classified according to their biochemical method of action (i.e., as alkylating agents, antimetabolites, antibiotics, or plant alkaloids). Examples of these agents and their mechanism of action are presented in Table 1-1.

Chemotherapy can be administered either as a single agent or as a combination of agents (e.g., an antimetabolite and an antibiotic). Currently, combination therapy is the most widely practiced protocol. Depending on the patient or the drug type, the agents may be given either orally or parenterally; parenteral

Table 1-1. Nonhormonal Cytotoxic Agents and Their Mechanism of Action

Drug	Agent Type	Mode of Action
Cyclophosphamide	Alkylating	Alkylation of hydrogen ions, resulting in interference with protein synthesis of DNA
Methotrexate	Antimetabolite	Inhibition of enzymatic activity, resulting in the disruption of DNA/RNA function
Bleomycin	Antibiotic	Direct inhibition of DNA/RNA function
Vincristine	Plant alkaloid	Alters microtubular assembly in mitotic spindle, causing metaphase arrest

administration involves intravenous, intramuscular, intrathecal, intracavitary, or intra-arterial infusion. Catheters, such as the Hickman or Broviac, are commonly used for frequent infusions. Those patients unable to tolerate multiple injections or who are unable to properly care for a catheter may require subcutaneous implantation of an injection port.

Hormones are often grouped under the classification of chemotherapy and include eight categories: estrogens, antiestrogens, progestins, androgens, antiandrogens, aromatase inhibitors, glucocorticoids, and gonadotropin-releasing hormone agonists.

It is imperative to keep in mind that the action of these chemotherapeutic drugs is not the direct killing of the tumor cells but a biochemical reaction that alters cell division and thereby cell proliferation.[31] The ultimate goal of chemotherapy is to inflict the greatest degree of damage to tumor cells at the least expense to normal cells and to the patient. Maximum benefit with acceptable morbidity determines the maximum tolerated dosage. Other factors associated with this decision include tumor type and grade; resistance/sensitivity; age, health, and well-being of the patient; and prognosis in terms of possible cure versus palliation.

Two major weaknesses inherent to chemotherapy are: (1) inability to prevent recurrence of disease; and (2) production of side effects commonly associated with cytotoxicity.

The most common side effect of various chemotherapeutic agents is myelosuppression. Reduction of the bone marrow's ability to produce sufficient life-sustaining cells can render the patient susceptible to opportunistic disease or even death. In addition to myelosuppression, the agents may have detrimental effects on organ systems, such as cardiac damage (anthracyclines), renal toxicity (high-dose methotrexate), pulmonary effects (bleomycin), hepatic toxicity (methotrexate), and neurologic damage (vincristine). Other less severe but common side effects include alopecia, mucositis, nausea and emesis, fatigue, and general malaise.

Controlled phases I to III research trials have provided a better understanding of the effect of chemotherapy on normal and malignant tissue. Many factors still require investigation in order to achieve the goal of maximum benefit and minimum morbidity. In the interim, patients will require strong support in psychosocial and emotional areas in order to maintain optimum quality of remaining life.

Radiation Therapy

Radiation therapy represents another antineoplastic method employed in the treatment of cancer. The process involves careful irradiation of tumor tissue by electromagnetic ionizing radiation. As with chemotherapy, its primary goal is to effect maximum tumor kill while maintaining acceptable levels of toxicity to normal surrounding tissue. Radiation therapy is generally used as either a curative or palliative strategy in the management of malignant neoplasms.

The evolution of radiation physics over the past century has been dramatic. Events such as World War II and recent nuclear accidents in the United States and abroad have accelerated the understanding of the effects of radiation on biologic tissue. Radiation therapy began in the early days with use of low-kilovoltage beams and progressed to high-kilovoltage ("soft") radiation of 200 to 400 kV.[32] This type of radiation often resulted in limited tumor kill and significant side effects, including excessive skin absorption, side scatter, and radiation sickness.

Since the late 1950s the development of megavoltage beams (1 to 25 Mev) has remarkably decreased the incidence of those side effects previously noted with low- or high-kilovoltage beams. Megavoltage radiation produced by either telecobalt units or linear accelerators results in the production of electromagnetic ionizing radiation streams consisting of x-rays, γ-rays, neutrons, and charged particles (protons and electrons). *Linear energy transfer* (LET) is the term associated with the amount of energy dissipated by the radiation beam as it passes through the absorbing tissue.[33] The higher the energy source the more radiation is absorbed at the deeper tissue levels. X-rays and γ-rays are examples of low LET radiation while neutrons are considered as exhibiting high LET characteristics.

Historically, *radiation absorbed dose* (rad) was the preferred term for describing the dose of ionizing radiation absorbed by the tissue—roughly 100 ergs/g.[32] Today, many radiation therapists prefer to use the term *centigrays* (cGy) instead of rad to identify the unit amount of radiation delivered to the tissue.

Relative biologic effect is a relatively new term used to express the biologic effectiveness of various types of ionizing radiation.[33] Its value is dependent on the site of radiation, the volume of tissue irradiated, the dose delivered, and the time in which radiation is delivered. Radiosensitivity of various biologic tissues is a critical factor to the effectiveness of radiation therapy. Cells that regularly divide and those with high oxygen content are considered radiosensitive and thus predictive of a favorable outcome; examples of such tissues include blood, intestinal villi, testes, and ovaries. Conversely, cells that are mature, divide slowly, or are of a hypoxic nature are significantly less sensitive and considered radioresistant; examples of such cells include those of bone (adult), nerves, muscles, and the endocrine system. Again, as in chemotherapy, the phase of the mammalian cell cycle is also critical to the effect of irradiation. Cells are most radiosensitive in the M/G2, G1/S, and S stages and are least sensitive in the late S and G0 stages.[34]

Method of Exposure

There are three main methods of administering radiation therapy: external beam (teletherapy), interstitial (brachytherapy), and intraoperative or intracavitary.

With external beam radiation, the most widely used method, the patient may be scheduled as an outpatient to receive a series of treatments to a localized area of the body over a period of 6 to 8 weeks. Typically, the first session involves a procedure known as *simulation,* in which the exact position, fields, and dosage are determined by the radiation therapist. Fluoroscopy and computer-assisted technology allow the therapist to consistently replicate the exact position and anticipated dosage for each session. The specific dosage varies in accordance with tumor size, extent, type, pathologic grade, differentiation, and level of radiosensitivity. *Fractionation* is the term applied to the frequency and dosage applied over time. For example, a breast cancer patient may be scheduled to receive 200 cGy 5 days a week for 6 to 8 weeks, for a total dose of 5,000 cGy.

Interstitial radiation (brachytherapy) involves implantation of radioactive material (i.e., seeds, wires, or solution) into the tumor bed for an initial period of 2 to 3 days.[35] During that time the patient is generally isolated in a special lead-lined hospital room and has minimal contact with family or medical personnel. The half-life of the radioactive substances used is short, and following their removal the patient is free to carry on with normal activities.

The third method of administration involves delivery of a high dose of radiation (via external beam) to a body cavity of the patient during an operative procedure. Intracavitary irradiation is sometimes the only method available to the surgeon or radiation oncologist for administering a life-preserving or life-lengthening dose of radiation.

Side Effects

A number of side effects may occur with any of these methods of treatment. Any or all of the biologic systems necessary for life may be affected in either the acute or chronic stage of the irradiation process. The two systems most critical to life involve the hematopoietic system and the gastrointestinal tract. Permanent dysfunction or infection involving these systems could result in a medical emergency and possible threat to the individual's life. Less severe but still very compromising are the side effects that involve other systems (e.g., cardiovascular, pulmonary, neurologic and musculoskeletal). Effects of radiation are typically classified according to the following four stages: acute (1 to 6 months), subacute (6 to 12 months), chronic (1 to 5 years), and late chronic (more than 5 years). The importance of these stages to the physical therapist becomes very evident during the course of treatment of these patients. For example, the breast cancer patient receiving radiation therapy following lumpectomy and axillary dissection may be discharged following her 6-week radiation treatment with full range of motion and no edema of the involved extremity. If not encouraged to continue with a program of stretching and elevation, the patient may return in 6 weeks with an adhesive capsulitis and significant edema of the extremity. The physiologic effect of radiation therapy does not end with the end of treatment but continues to show changes on a microcellular level for 6 months to 1 year. Adhesions involving the collagen matrix of connective tissue and fibrosis of vasculature and lymphatics are not atypical at 1 year.

Radiation therapy has made great strides in the perfection of its administration and dosage techniques owing in part to changes in technology and also to the level of professional expertise developed by these radiology technicians over the last few decades. A close relationship between the radiation oncologist and the physical therapist is necessary in order to bring about the most functional and pain-free outcome for many patients undergoing radiation therapy.

Immunotherapy

Immunotherapy is the newest and most promising medical strategy being investigated and in some cases implemented in the treatment of cancer. The term associated with this class of agents is *biologic response modifier.* Initial investigational studies in this area began in the late 1950s with the bacterial strain *Mycobacterium bovis.* The specific agent produced was named bacillus Calmette-Guérin and was originally used for immunization against tuberculosis. It was later discovered to exhibit immunogenic properties consistent with tumor regression.[36] Since that time a number of different biologic response modifiers have been identified and are currently undergoing in vitro and in vivo investigation. An excellent review of these agents and their investigative studies is available in an article by Lotze and Rosenberg on immunologic treatment of cancer.[37]

Currently, alpha interferon is the only biologic response modifier that has received approval from the Food and Drug Administration for commercial use. Each agent varies in description, action, and side effects (Table 1-2), the main objective of each being either direct or indirect tumor kill through bolstering of the body's natural immune system.

As mentioned, the area of immunotherapy is new but holds much promise

Table 1-2. Common Biologic Response Modifiers

Agent	Description	Action	Common Side Effects
Bacillus Calmette-Guérin	Strain of *Mycobacterium bovis*	Complex: may involve stimulation of lymphocytes and macrophages	Bladder and urinary dysfunction, influenza-like symptoms
Interferon ([a] α-, β-, and γ-gamma)	Group of proteins and glycoproteins	Antiviral, immuno-modulatory, and antiproliferative	High fever, chills, malaise, fatigue, weakness, and weight loss
Interleukin (IL-2, IL-4)	Lymphokine produced by T lymphocytes	Antiproliferation, enhancement of T-cell production	Capillary permeability leak syndrome: fluid retention, weight gain
Monoclonal antibodies	Product of immune β lymphocytes	Immune-mediated destruction, antiproliferation, cytotoxic effect	Chills, fever, flushing, nausea, vomiting, skin rashes
Tumor necrosis factor	Glycoprotein	Cytotoxic effect	

[a] Only biologic response modifier approved by the Food and Drug Administration to be used in the treatment of cancer (hairy-cell leukemia). All other agents listed are considered investigational agents currently undergoing investigational trials.

and may be the least invasive method by which one can produce an antineoplastic effect at minimal cost to the host. The most common side effect that the physical therapist may need to address in patients treated by this method may be cardiovascular and metabolic deficits subsequent to fluid retention and immobilization. Edema, weakness, pain, and decreased endurance may be among the problem areas requiring the most intervention.

REFERENCES

1. Sondik EJ, Young JL, Horm JW, Gloeckler-Ries LA: Annual Cancer Statistics Review. U.S. Department of Health and Human Services, Public Health Service, National Institutes of Health, National Cancer Institute, Bethesda. NIH Publication No. 89-2789, 1988
2. Sondik EJ, Kessler LG, Gloeckler-Ries LA: Cancer Statistics Review 1973–1986. U.S. Department of Health and Human Services, Public Health Service, National Institutes of Health, National Cancer Institute, Bethesda. NIH Publication No. 89-2789, May 1989
3. Cancer Facts and Figures. American Cancer Society, Atlanta, 1989
4. Gerber LH, McGarvey CL: Musculoskeletal deficits and rehabilitation intervention in the cancer patient. pp. 579–582. In Wittes RE (ed): Manual of Oncologic Therapeutics 1989/1990. JB Lippincott, Philadelphia, 1989
5. MacMahon HE: The pathology of malignancy. p. 15. In Cancer—A Manual for Practitioners, 4th Ed. American Cancer Society, Atlanta, 1968

6. Bonfiglio TA, Terry R: The pathology of cancer, p. 20. In Rubin P (ed): Clinical Oncology: A Multidisciplinary Approach. 6th Ed. American Cancer Society, Atlanta, 1983
7. DeVita VT: Cancer Treatment and Medicine for the Layman. U.S. Dept of Health and Human Services. Public Health Service, National Institutes of Health, Bethesda, 1977
8. Baserga R: The cell cycle. N Engl J Med 304:453, 1981
9. Pardee AB: Principles of cancer biology: Cell biology and biochemistry of cancer. p. 59. In DeVita VT, Hellman S, Rosenberg SA (eds): Cancer: Principles and Practices of Oncology. JB Lippincott, Philadelphia, 1982
10. Hill HZ, Lin HS: Carcinogenesis and tumor growth. p. 1. In Horton J, Hill GJ (eds): Clinical Oncology. WB Saunders, Philadelphia, 1977
11. Kempson RL, Hendrickson MR: The impact of pathology on cancer treatment. p. 26. In Carter SK, Glatstein E, Livingston RB (eds): Principles of Cancer Treatment. McGraw-Hill, New York, 1982
12. Terry R: Pathology of cancer. p. 11. In Rubin P (ed): Clinical Oncology, 5th Ed. American Cancer Society, Atlanta, 1978
13. Upton AC: Principles of cancer biology: Etiology and prevention of cancer. p. 33. In DeVita VT, Hellman S, Rosenberg SA (eds): Cancer: Principles and Practices of Oncology. JB Lippincott, Philadelphia, 1982
14. Bakemeier RF: Basic concepts of cancer chemotherapy and principles of medical oncology. p. 82. In Rubin P (ed): Clinical Oncology: A Multidisciplinary Approach 6th Ed. American Cancer Society, Atlanta, 1983
15. Harris J: Tumor immunology. p. 192. In Horton J, Hill GJ (eds): Clinical Oncology. WB Saunders, Philadelphia, 1977
16. Merigan TC: Virology and immune mechanisms. Cancer 47:1091, 1981
17. Morton DL, Goodnight J: Cancer immunology and immunotherapy. p. 124. In Haskell CK (ed): Cancer Treatment. WB Saunders, Philadelphia, 1980
18. Shimkin MB: Research on the causes and nature of cancer. p. 1. In del Regato JA, Spjut HJ, Cox JD (eds): Ackerman and del Regato's Cancer, Diagnosis, Treatment, and Prognosis. CV Mosby, St Louis, 1985
19. Commission on Clinical Oncology of the Union Internationale Contre le Cancer [International Union Against Cancer (UICC)]: TNM Classification of Malignant Tumours. International Union Against Cancer, Geneva, 1968
20. Beahrs OH, Henson DE, Hutter RVP, Myers MH (eds): American Joint Committee on Cancer (AJCC) Manual for Staging of Cancer. 3rd Ed. JB Lippincott, Philadelphia, 1988
21. Rubin P: Statement of the clinical oncologic problem. p. 2. In Rubin P (ed): Clinical Oncology: A Multidisciplinary Approach. 6th Ed. American Cancer Society, Atlanta, 1983
22. McKenna RJ Jr, McKenna RJ: Overview of surgical oncology. p. 3. In McKenna RJ, Murphy GP (eds): Fundamentals of Surgical Oncology. Macmillan, New York, 1986
23. Pilch YH (ed): Surgical Oncology. McGraw-Hill, New York, 1984
24. Rosenberg SA: Principles of surgical oncology. p. 215. In DeVita VT, Hellman S, Rosenberg SA (eds): Cancer Principles and Practice of Oncology. Vol. 2. JB Lippincott, Philadelphia, 1985
25. Patterson WB: Principles of surgical oncology. p. 30. In Rubin P (ed): Clinical Oncology: A Multidisciplinary Approach. 6th Ed. American Cancer Society, Atlanta, 1983

26. McKenna RJ, Murphy GP (eds): Fundamentals of Surgical Oncology. MacMillan, New York, 1986
27. DeVita VT, Hellman S, Rosenberg SA (eds): Cancer Principles and Practice of Oncology. 3rd Ed. JB Lippincott, Philadelphia, 1989
28. O'Connel TX: Surgical Oncology: Controversies in Cancer Treatment. G.K. Hall Medical Publishers, Boston, 1981
29. Rosenberg SA (ed): Surgical Treatment of Metastatic Cancer. JB Lippincott, Philadelphia, 1987
30. Wittes RE, Jones-Leyland B, Fortner C, Hubband SM: Chemotherapy: The properties and uses of single agents. p. 91. In Wittes RE (ed): Manual of Oncologic Therapeutics 1989/1990. JB Lippincott, Philadelphia, 1989
31. Carter SK, Bakowski MT, Hellman K: Basic concepts in cancer chemotherapy. p. 9. In Carter SK (ed): Chemotherapy of Cancer. 3rd Ed. Churchill Livingstone, New York, 1987
32. Keller BE, Rubin P: Basic concepts of radiation physics. p. 72. In Rubin P (ed): Clinical Oncology: A Multidisciplinary Approach. 6th Ed. American Cancer Society, Atlanta, 1983
33. Sutherland RM, Mulcahy RT: Basic principles of radiation biology. p. 40. In Rubin P (ed): Clinical Oncology: A Multidisciplinary Approach. 6th Ed. American Cancer Society, Atlanta, 1983
34. Rubin P: Principles of radiation oncology and cancer radiotherapy. p. 59. In Rubin P (ed): Clinical Oncology: A Multidisciplinary Approach. 6th Ed. American Cancer Society, Atlanta, 1983
35. Shank B: Radiotherapy: Implications for general patient care. p. 89. In Wittes RE (ed): Manual of Oncologic Therapeutics 1989/1990. JB Lippincott, Philadelphia, 1989
36. Krown SE: Biologic response modifiers. p. 178. In Wittes RE (ed): Manual of Oncologic Therapeutics 1989/1990. JB Lippincott, Philadelphia, 1989
37. Lotze MT, Rosenberg SA: The immunologic treatment of cancer. CA 38:69, 1988

Appendices

Appendix 1-1. Glossary

Adenocarcinoma	A form of cancer that involves the cells lining the walls of many different glandular organs in the body.
Alkylating agents	Anticancer drugs that substitute an alkyl group for an active hydrogen atom in an organic compound (e.g., cyclophosphamide).
Alopecia	Loss of hair.
Anaplasia	A loss of differentiation of cells and of their orientation to one another, a characteristic of tumor tissue.
Antibiotics	Anticancer drugs that bind to DNA and inhibit DNA and RNA synthesis (e.g., Adriamycin).
Antimetabolites	Anticancer drugs that interfere with the processes of DNA production and thus prevent cell division (e.g., methotrexate).
Antineoplastic therapy	Procedures employed to control or terminate neoplastic processes. These include surgery, chemotherapy, radiation therapy, immunotherapy, and hormonal therapy.
CT	Computed tomography.
Cachexia	A profound and marked state of constitutional disorder; general ill health and malnutrition.
Cancer	A general term for a large group of diseases (more than 100), all characterized by uncontrolled growth and spread of abnormal cells.
Carcinoma	A form of cancer arising from epithelial tissue. It develops in tissues covering or lining organs of the body, such as skin, the uterus, the lung, or the breast.
Carcinoma in situ	An early stage in development when the cancer is still confined to the tissues of origin. In situ carcinomas are highly curable.
Chemotherapy	Use of chemical substances alone or in combination to control or palliate cancer processes. These include antimetabolites, alkylating agents, antibiotics, vinca alkaloids, and hormones.
Hormone and Hormone Inhibitors	Estrogens, androgens, progestins, adrenocorticosteroids, and antiestrogens.
Hyperplasia	An abnormal multiplication or increase in number of normal cells in normal arrangement in a tissue.
Immunotherapy	Use of biological response modifiers, a new class of compounds such as interferon, which fight cancer by stimulating the body's immune system.
Incidence	The extent to which disease occurs in the population. Cancer incidence is the estimated number of new cases of cancer diagnosed per year.
Leukopenia	Decrease in the number of leukocytes (white blood cells).
Limb Salvage/Limb Sparing	Conservative surgical technique to remove primary tumor from an extremity.
Metastasis	The spread of cancer cells to distant areas of the body by way of the lymph system or bloodstream.

(continued)

Appendix 1-1. Glossary (*continued*)

Mitosis	Process of cell production—cell division in four phases.
Monoclonal antibodies	Antibodies designed to seek out chosen targets on cancer cells. They are under study for possible delivery of chemotherapy and radiotherapy directly to a cancer, thus killing the cancerous cell and sparing healthy tissue. Studies are also underway to determine if monoclonal antibodies can be produced that will detect and diagnose cancer cells at a very early curable stage.
Morbidity	Sickness. The term refers to the proportion of people with an illness.
Mortality	Death. Mortality rates reflect the number of deaths in a given population.
NMR/MRI	Nuclear magnetic resonance; magnetic resonance imaging.
Neoplasm	Any new abnormal growth. Neoplasms may be benign or malignant, but the term is generally used to describe a cancer.
Oncology	The science dealing with the physical, chemical, and biologic properties and features of cancer, including causes and the disease process.
Palliation therapy	Therapy that relieves symptoms, such as pain, but does not alter the course of the disease. Its primary purpose is to improve the quality of life.
PET	Positron emission tomography.
Pleomorphism	The assumption of various distinct forms by a single organism or species.
Prevalence	The number of patients with a disease in the population at a specific time. For example, the prevalence of esophageal cancer is higher in blacks than in whites.
Radiotherapy	Treatment with high-energy radiation. Radiation therapy may be used to reduce the size of a cancer before surgery or to destroy any remaining cancer after surgery. Radiotherapy can be helpful in shrinking recurrent cancers to relieve symptoms. Examples include intraoperative radiation (IR), external beam radiation (ER), and radioactive implants.
Recurrence (local)	Reappearance of cancer after a disease-free period.
Relapse	Reappearance of cancer after a disease-free period.
Remission	Complete or partial disappearance of the signs and symptoms of disease in response to treatment. The period during which a disease is under control. A remission does not necessarily indicate a cure.
Sarcoma	A form of cancer arising from nonepithelial (mesenchymal) tissue, including bone, cartilage, fat, or muscle.
Staging	An evaluation of the extent of a disease such as cancer. A classification based on stage at diagnosis helps determine appropriate treatment and prognosis.
Thrombocytopenia	Decrease in the number of cell platelets.
Vinca alkaloids	Anticancer drugs that interfere with microtubule assembly in mitotic spindle formation (e.g., vincristine).

Appendix 1-2. Cancer Resources

Agency	Address and Phone Numbers	Resources
American Cancer Society National Local	1599 Clifton Rd., N.E. Atlanta, GA 30329 404-320-3333 800-4-CANCER (U.S.) Alaska 800-638-6070 Washington DC & suburbs 202-636-5700 Hawaii 524-1234	Public Education Materials Health Professionals Education Materials Facts & Figures Reach To Recovery Cansurmount I CAN COPE
National Cancer Institute (NCI)	National Cancer Institute Public Inquiries National Institutes of Health Bldg. 10-A, Room 24 9000 Rockville Pike Bethesda, MD 20892 301-496-5583	Public Education Materials Health Professional Education Materials
American Physical Therapy Association (APTA)	1111 N. Fairfax Street Alexandria, VA 22314 703-684-2782; 800-999-2782	Bibliography on cancer articles
APTA Section on Oncology (Section of the APTA, Inc.)	Name, address, and number of section president may be obtained by calling the APTA at 800-999-2782 (Component Relations)	Membership in section Bibliography Continuing education
U.S. Dept. of Health & Human Services, Public Health Service, National Institutes of Health Bethesda, MD 20205	Biometry Branch, Division of Cancer Prevention and Control, National Cancer Institute 301-496-5583	SEER Program: Cancer Incidence and Mortality in the United States, NIH Publication #89-1837; 1986 Annual Cancer Statistics Review, NIH Publication #89-2789
U.S. Dept. of Health & Human Services, Public Health Service, National Center for Health Statistics	3700 East-West Highway Hyattsville, MD 20782 301-436-8500	Monthly vital statistics report Mortality rates
National Library of Medicine	8600 Rockville Pike Bethesda, MD 20892 301-496-4000	International Cancer Research Data Base (ICRDB) Physicians Desk Query (PDQ) Medical Cancerlit database
National Coalition Cancer Survivorship	323 Eighth Street, S.W. Albuquerque, NM 87102 505-764-9956	Clearinghouse for publication of cancer survivors
MAKE TODAY COUNT	P.O. Box 222 Osage Beach, MO 65065	Newsletter Emotional support to persons with cancer

(*continued*)

Appendix 1-2. Cancer Resources (*continued*)

Agency	Address and Phone Numbers	Resources
Operation Uplift	1703 W. 14th Port Angeles, WA 98362	Support for breast cancer patients
Art That Heals	Johnsson Cancer Center, UCLA Louis Factor Building 10-247 10883 LeConte Avenue Los Angeles, CA 90024	Posters and art catalogue produced by artists who are cancer survivors

2 | Rehabilitation of the Lung Cancer Patient

Bernadette D. Shea
Georgann Vlad

Lung cancer is a significant health problem in the United States—in 1988 an estimated 152,000 new cases were diagnosed and 139,000 deaths were attributed to the disease.[1] Lung cancer has become the most common cause of cancer deaths among both men and women.[1] Cigarette smoking is the leading cause of lung cancer in the United States.[2] Environmental risk factors include exposure to asbestos dust, arsenic, chromium, nickel, chloromethyl ethers, and vinyl chloride.[3]

The vast majority of lung cancers arise from the epithelium of the bronchial and bronchioalveolar surfaces and from the bronchial mucous glands. Epithelial carcinomas are generally classified into one of four cell types: squamous cell carcinoma, adenocarcinoma, large cell carcinoma, and small cell carcinoma. Squamous cell (epidermoid) carcinomas typically arise centrally, although they may arise in peripheral lung tissue as well. These tumors tend to invade the bronchial wall, adjoining lung tissue, pulmonary vessels, and lymph nodes. Adenocarcinomas usually arise more peripherally but may be found centrally. These tumors invade the pleura, hilar or mediastinal lymph nodes, and cardiovascular system. Early distant metastases, notably to the brain, liver, bone, and central nervous system, are common. Most large cell carcinomas are peripheral in origin. These tumors are relatively large in size and invade local lung tissue and surrounding pleura. Distant metastasis occurs late in the disease course.

Small cell carcinoma typically arises centrally and has the strongest correlation with cigarette smoking. These tumors grow rapidly, and early invasion of adjoining bronchial, mediastinal, and hilar lymph nodes is common, approximately 70 percent of patients showing extensive disease at the time of diagnosis.[4] Because of the early and widespread metastasis of small cell carcinoma, it carries the gravest prognosis as compared with other histologic types of lung cancer, from which it also differs in terms of disease course and treatment. Therefore, a distinction is generally made between small cell lung cancer (SCLC) and non-small cell lung cancer (NSCLC).

Generally, symptomatic lung cancer is indicative of advanced disease, although presymptomatic disease does not necessarily correspond to an early stage. Survival rates tend to be better when the tumor is small, localized, and asymptomatic.[5] Symptoms of lung cancer include chronic cough, dyspnea, chest pain, hemoptysis, and wheezing.

A variety of diagnostic measures are available to detect lung cancer. In addition to chest radiographs and sputum cytology, fiberoptic bronchoscopy is useful in supplying cytologic material. Percutaneous needle aspiration biopsy is another important diagnostic technique and involves minimal discomfort for the patient. Computed tomography (CT) is helpful in delineating the extent of tumor involvement in the lung and mediastinum. Mediastinoscopy is performed to obtain further tissue diagnosis from mediastinal nodes.

NON-SMALL CELL LUNG CANCER
Staging

Staging of lung cancer assesses the extent of tumor involvement in a patient at the time of diagnosis. This information is quite valuable for making therapeutic decisions and prognostic predictions. The information sought in assigning a stage includes tumor size and location, extent of tumor invasion, and the presence of regional or metastatic disease.

The need for a standardized staging system for lung cancer was recognized by the Task Force on Lung Cancer of the American Joint Committee on Cancer Staging and End Results Reporting (AJCC),[6] which developed a system based on the TNM system first put forth by Denoix.[7] Recently the classification system was modified to provide a new international staging system developed by the Task Force on Lung Cancer of the AJCC in cooperation with the International Union Against Cancer. In 1985 this new staging system (Table 2-1) was presented by Mountain at the Fourth World Conference on Lung Cancer.[8]

In the TNM staging system T represents the primary tumor, with subscripts indicating its size or the extent of local invasion; N represents regional lymph nodes, with subscripts indicating the extent of nodal involvement; and M represents distant metastatic disease, with subscripts indicating the presence or absence of such spread. Once a case has received a TNM classification, it is further assigned to the appropriate stage in the international staging system (Table 2-2).

Stage I lung cancer includes tumors confined to the lung with no lymph node

Table 2-1. TNM Definitions

TX	A tumor proven by the presence of malignant cells in bronchopulmonary secretions but not visualized radiographically or bronchoscopically or any tumor that cannot be assessed, as in a retreatment staging.
T0	No evidence of primary tumor.
Tis	Carcinoma in situ.
T1	A tumor that is 3.0 cm or less in greatest dimension, surrounded by lung or visceral pleura, and without evidence of invasion proximal to a lobar bronchus at bronchoscopy.[a]
T2	A tumor more than 3.0 cm in greatest dimension or a tumor of any size that either invades the visceral pleura or has associated atelectasis or obstructive pneumonitis extending to the hilar region. At bronchoscopy the proximal extent of demonstrable tumor must be within a lobar bronchus or at least 2.0 cm distal to the carina. Any associated atelectasis or obstructive pneumonitis must involve less than an entire lung.
T3	A tumor of any size with direct extension into the chest wall (including superior sulcus tumors), diaphragm, or the mediastinal pleura or pericardium without involving the heart, great vessels, trachea, esophagus, or vertebral body, or a tumor in the main bronchus within 2 cm of the carina without involving the carina.
T4	A tumor of any size with invasion of the mediastinum; with involvement of the heart, great vessels, trachea, esophagus, vertebral body, or carina; or accompanied by malignant pleural effusion.[b]
N0	No demonstrable metastasis to regional lymph nodes.
N1	Metastasis to lymph nodes in the peribronchial region, the ipsilateral hilar region, or both, including direct extension.
N2	Metastasis to ipsilateral mediastinal lymph nodes and subcarinal lymph nodes.
N3	Metastasis to contralateral mediastinal lymph nodes, contralateral hilar lymph nodes, or ipsilateral or contralateral scalene or supraclavicular lymph nodes.
M0	No (known) distant metastasis.
M1	Distant metastasis present.

[a] The uncommon superficial tumor of any size having its invasive component limited to the bronchial wall and possibly extending proximal to the main bronchus is classified as T1.

[b] Most pleural effusions associated with lung cancer are due to tumor. There are, however, some few patients in whom cytopathologic examination of pleural fluid (on more than one specimen) is negative for tumor and whose fluid is nonbloody and is not an exudate. In such cases, in which these elements and clinical judgment dictate that the effusion is not related to the tumor, patients should be staged as T1, T2 or T3, with exclusion of effusion as a staging element. (From Mountain,[8] with permission.)

involvement and no distant metastasis. Stage II disease includes T1 or T2 tumors with involvement of the peribronchial, lobar, or hilar lymph nodes. Stage III tumors are advanced lung cancers confined to the thorax. This category is subdivided into two substages, IIIa and IIIb. Stage IIIa includes T3N0 and T3N1 disease, as well as T1 to T3 tumors with metastasis limited to the

Table 2-2. Stage Grouping of TNM Subsets

Occult carcinoma	TX N0 M0
Stage 0	Tis—carcinoma in situ
Stage I	T1 N0 M0
	T2 N0 M0
Stage II	T1 N1 M0
	T2 N1 M0
Stage IIIa	T3 N0 M0
	T3 N1 M0
	T1–3 N2 M0
Stage IIIb	Any T N3 M0
	T4 Any N M0
Stage IV	Any T any N M1

(From Mountain,[8] with permission.)

ipsilateral mediastinal and subcarinal lymph nodes. Stage IIIb lung cancer includes any tumor that is more extensive than T3, any tumor with metastasis to supraclavicular, scalene, or contralateral mediastinal and hilar lymph nodes, or any tumor with a malignant pleural effusion. Stage IV disease includes any lung tumor presenting with distant metastasis.

Treatment

Treatment of lung cancer includes surgery, radiation therapy, chemotherapy, and often some combination of these modalities. The treatment approach is dependent on the histology of the tumor and the degree of invasion and metastasis at the time of diagnosis, as well as the overall medical condition of the patient.

Surgery

A patient with NSCLC may be considered a candidate for surgical intervention if the tumor is localized and contained within an area where it can be safely excised. The patient's cardiac and pulmonary functional status must also be considered. Patients with stage I and II disease are generally considered to be potential surgical candidates. Successful surgical intervention in patients with stage III disease is dependent on a number of factors. T3 tumors without nodal involvement have the best prognosis, the potential for successful resection of such tumors depending upon the area or organ invaded. Invasion of the major vessels, diaphragm, or vertebral bodies corresponds to a poor prognosis.[9] Stage IV disease is generally not considered to be resectable, but in some cases patients with completely resectable lung disease and a solitary brain metastasis may undergo surgical resection of both the lung and brain lesions. Magilligan et al. report a 25 percent 5-year survival rate with this approach.[10]

The location and extent of disease will determine the surgical procedure undertaken. Regional lymph nodes must be removed and examined for evidence of disease. A *wedge resection,* or *segmentectomy,* may be performed when patients are unable to tolerate a more extensive resection owing to their poor functional status or general medical condition. In these cases a wedge resection of peripheral T1 or T2 tumors may be performed, thereby preserving as much lung tissue as possible. There is some debate as to whether this procedure is as effective in treating T1N0 and T2N0 disease as is a lobectomy.[11,12]

A lobectomy is performed when the tumor can be excised without removing the entire lung. A *pneumonectomy* is performed when the tumor occurs proximally and complete resection does not allow conservation of lung tissue. *Sleeve pneumonectomy* involves removal of tumor that invades the proximal main stem bronchus and possibly the carina itself. This procedure is performed infrequently and only in very select instances since the associated morbidity and mortality can be prohibitive.

A carcinoma that has invaded the chest wall requires resection of the affected lung and chest wall. Resultant large chest wall defects are reconstructed with plastic mesh. Smaller chest wall defects may not require reconstruction.

Radiotherapy

Radiotherapy as a Primary Treatment Modality. In most cases patients with NSCLC who receive radiation therapy as a primary treatment modality have unresectable intrathoracic disease. This group has a 5-year survival rate of approximately 5 percent.[13–15]

The role of radiotherapy as a primary treatment modality in cases of potentially resectable disease is controversial since radiation is viewed as less effective than surgery. The major limiting factor in determining whether or not radiotherapy can be delivered in curative doses is the patient's pulmonary function. Patients with limited pulmonary reserve receive limited doses of radiation in an effort to preserve as much uninvolved lung tissue as possible.

Preoperative Adjuvant Radiotherapy. The use of preoperative radiotherapy has been investigated, particularly with respect to its ability to shrink unresectable tumors to resectable size. With the exception of superior sulcus tumors, preoperative adjuvant radiotherapy has not been found to be beneficial in terms of increased survival in patients with NSCLC.[16–18] Paulson has reported significant benefit of preoperative radiotherapy in superior sulcus tumors.[19]

Postoperative Adjuvant Radiotherapy. Although postoperative radiotherapy has been widely used in cases of locally invasive lung cancer for years, no firm evidence of its benefit in terms of long-term survival has been demonstrated. Several studies have shown postoperative radiotherapy to be effective in local control of squamous carcinoma.[20,21] The Lung Cancer Study Group, in a study of patients with stage II and stage III squamous carcinoma of the lung,[21] reported a 3 percent incidence of local recurrence in the group treated with postoperative radiotherapy and a 35 percent incidence of recurrence in the control group. They were unable to demonstrate a significant difference in survival between the two groups. At present postoperative radiotherapy in disease with no nodal involvement is not generally recommended.[22–24]

Radiation Therapy as a Palliative Measure. Radiotherapy has been demonstrated to be effective in relieving symptoms of lung cancer patients, including hemoptysis, chest pain, superior vena cava syndrome, and dyspnea.[25] Palliative radiotherapy is generally administered at a lower dose in an effort to conserve as much healthy lung tissue as possible.

Interstitial Radiation. Intraoperative brachytherapy is delivered via implantation of radioactive seeds or afterloading catheters at the time of thoracotomy. This procedure allows delivery of a higher dose of radiation than is possible with external radiation. In studies at Memorial Sloan-Kettering Cancer Center radioactive sources were directly inserted into the tumor, permitting a more localized effect of irradiation.[26] The radiation dose falls off rapidly outside the tumor, which results in less damage to surrounding healthy tissue.

In a recent review of patients treated with brachytherapy at Memorial Sloan-Kettering Cancer Center, Hilaris and Martini reported that brachytherapy, used in combination with surgery and postoperative external radiation, improved local control of disease in advanced cases and that a slight improvement in survival could be demonstrated.[27] Further study of this approach in the treatment of lung cancer is needed.

Chemotherapy

The majority of patients diagnosed with NSCLC either initially present with or later develop metastatic disease.[28,29] Thus, there is great interest in chemotherapy as a systemic treatment approach in this group of patients. The preferred method of treatment is to use a combination of drugs rather than single agents.[30] The role of combination chemotherapy in the treatment of recurrent and metastatic NSCLC remains the subject of some debate.[31,32]

It has been demonstrated that those patients who respond to combination chemotherapy will do so within 6 to 12 weeks from initiation of therapy.[33] Patients with a good performance status generally have a better response to treatment.[34] Further, a better response rate is observed in patients with intrathoracic disease than in patients with widely disseminated disease.[35,36] Still, few unresectable patients with NSCLC who are treated with combination chemotherapy alone survive longer than 30 months.[37–39] Further randomized clinical trials are needed to demonstrate what effect, if any, combination chemotherapy has on long-term survival.

Radiation and Chemotherapy

The possible benefits of administering combination chemotherapy and radiotherapy in an effort to control both local and systemic disease has been the subject of much study.[40–42] As of 1989 there is no firm evidence to demonstrate that long-term survival is improved by combining chemotherapy and radiotherapy.[43]

Combination Chemotherapy, Radiotherapy and Surgery

The use of preoperative chemotherapy with or without radiotherapy in NSCLC is under investigation. Takita and colleagues have reported on their experience in treating 24 inoperable NSCLC patients with this multimodal approach[44]; 20 of their patients were alive at 27 months, while the other 4 died without evidence of disease.

In a pilot study conducted at Rush-Presbyterian-St. Luke's Medical Center, patients with advanced NSCLC were treated with preoperative combination chemotherapy, radiotherapy, and surgery.[45] Of the 39 patients who subsequently underwent surgery, 9 patients (23 percent) were found to be histologically tumor-free, 8 patients (21 percent) had microscopic residual disease, and 22 patients (56 percent) were found to have gross residual tumor. Median survival for the group was 20 months.

In a 1988 report by Martini and colleagues on 41 NSCLC patients with N2M0 disease who were treated with preoperative chemotherapy, 30 patients (73 percent) demonstrated a significant radiographic response to the treatment; 28 of these patients subsequently underwent thoracotomy, 21 of whom (75 percent) had a complete resection of disease, while 4 patients presented with limited microscopic foci of residual tumor. Of those patients who underwent chemotherapy and surgery, 40 percent were alive 3 years from the time of diagnosis.[46]

While early results of this multimodal approach to treating NSCLC are encouraging, it remains unclear whether this approach is more successful in terms of survival than treatment by surgery or radiation alone. Further studies are currently underway to ascertain the benefit of this investigational multimodality treatment.

SMALL CELL LUNG CANCER

SCLC differs from NSCLC, in terms of both disease course and response to radiotherapy and chemotherapeutic agents. The disease is marked by rapid growth and early development of distant metastases.[47] The majority of patients with SCLC present with disseminated disease,[48,49] and those who are untreated have median survivals of 6 to 17 weeks.[50,51]

Staging

The TNM staging system is less useful in SCLC than in NSCLC, since more than 95 percent of patients will be classified as stage III.[52] Most investigators use a two-stage system introduced by the American Veterans Administration Lung Cancer Study, which classifies patients as having either limited or extensive disease.[50] *Limited disease* is defined as disease confined to one hemithorax, with or without involvement of the supraclavicular nodes. *Extensive disease* refers to tumor outside these boundaries.

Treatment of Small Cell Lung Cancer

Despite years of investigative study, the optimal treatment of SCLC remains in question. Prior to 1970 surgery and radiation therapy were the most common forms of treatment offered to these patients. Long-term survival rates were extremely poor.[53-55] Recognition of the early metastasis in this disease has since shifted the emphasis to systemic chemotherapy.

Chemotherapy

SCLC is markedly sensitive to chemotherapy, and most tumors will respond to such therapy initially. In fact, approximately 30 to 40 percent of patients with limited disease and 15 to 20 percent of patients with extensive disease will respond completely to combination chemotherapy.[52] It appears that those patients who respond completely to initial therapeutic intervention do better overall than partial responders.[56] Unfortunately, the duration of response is often short, and most patients will relapse.[47] The majority of these tumors quickly become resistant to drug therapy, and following initial treatment failure, tumor response to secondary chemotherapeutic agents is of short duration, if achieved at all.[47]

The optimal duration of therapy has not been defined. Several studies report the efficacy of short intensive courses of chemotherapy.[57-59] Many patients who achieve a complete response do so in the first 6 weeks of chemotherapy.[60] As of 1988 most patients receive first-line combination chemotherapy for 6 months to 1 year.[52,61] Maintenance chemotherapy has not been shown to be useful in increasing long-term survival.[62] Drug combinations, dosage, and frequency and duration of treatment remain controversial.

Radiation Therapy

Small cell carcinoma is the most radiosensitive of all lung cancers.[52] Studies have shown, however, that patients with limited disease treated with radiotherapy alone have poor survival rates.[63,64] Moreover, the chest is a site of failure in a significant number of patients with limited disease.[55] The question thus arises as to the merits of combining chemotherapy and radiotherapy. Radiotherapy has been shown to decrease the incidence of local recurrence,[65] but a combination of chemotherapy and radiotherapy has not been shown to be more effective in terms of median survival than chemotherapy alone.[52] The most effective method of combining these modalities remains under investigation, as does their effect on long-term survival.

Prophylactic Cranial Irradiation in Small Cell Lung Cancer. It is estimated that of those patients with SCLC who survive 2 years, 80 percent will develop brain metastases without preventive measures.[66] Administration of chemotherapeutic agents that cross the blood-brain barrier do not appear to change these statistics.[66] A number of nonrandomized studies have shown that the incidence of brain metastases is significantly reduced with prophylactic cranial irradiation.[48,55] The question that remains is whether such irradiation has a significant effect on long-term survival. This is of particular concern in view of the potentially severe side effects of cranial irradiation.

Surgery

A surgical approach in the treatment of SCLC was generally abandoned in the 1970s following a number of studies that showed no long-term survivors among patients treated by surgery.[54,67] However, interest in this area has been renewed in the 1980s by encouraging results of a number of studies.[68–71] In a study performed by the Veterans Administration Surgical Oncology Group, 148 patients with SCLC who underwent potentially curative resection were randomized to one of four prospective adjuvant chemotherapy trials.[72] Based on 5-year survival rates, the study concluded that surgical resection was indicated in patients with T1 N0 M0 disease and possibly in those with T1 N1 M0 and T2 N0 M0 disease. Additionally, it was reported that surgery is contraindicated in all other TNM categories.

Despite improvements in the treatment of SCLC, the majority of patients die from their disease. Median survival rates in patients with limited disease are between 12 and 16 months,[48,73] and patients with extensive disease have median survival rates between 7 and 12 months.[48,73] Overall, only 4 percent of patients with SCLC survive beyond 5 years.[61]

PHYSICAL THERAPY INTERVENTION

While the medical management of lung cancer often involves the triad of surgery, chemotherapy, and/or radiation therapy, the surgical patient presents with common problems that necessitate physical therapy intervention. Whether the surgical procedure is a lobectomy, pneumonectomy, or segmental or sleeve resection, the following physical therapy program can serve as a guideline for management of the surgical lung cancer patient.

Physical therapy problems usually associated with the surgical patient include an ineffective and unproductive cough, decreased chest expansion, poor breathing ratio, decreased trunk mobility, decreased ambulation tolerance, and pain. Appropriate short- and long-term goals for the above problems include: demonstration of an effective and productive cough; return to preoperative chest expansion in proportion to extent of lung resected; demonstration of appropriate breathing ratio; return to preoperative trunk mobility status; ambulation tolerance of 1,000 feet on level terrain with no or appropriate shortness of breath; and resolution or management of pain.[74]

Ideally, the patient is referred for physical therapy evaluation prior to surgery. This initial contact allows for patient education and instruction and for obtaining baseline measurements. The components of this initial evaluation include a standard chart review, with emphasis on current disease state, prior medical control, planned medical management, and reason for admission. Laboratory findings should be reviewed to establish baseline information, including pulmonary function tests; arterial blood gases; electrocardiogram; blood chemistry; results of scans such as bone scan, CT scan, or magnetic resonance imaging (MRI); results of mediastinoscopy; and conventional radiographic findings.

The subjective portion of the evaluation may present some obstacles (e.g., denial and fear) not frequently encountered to the same degree in the noncancer patient. It is essential to understand patients' perception of the disease, along with their specific knowledge base in order to establish mutually realistic goals. Information regarding the family structure will help to identify a primary caregiver (if one exists) who can provide both physical and emotional support. Financial status and employment history can provide insight into decision making. Exposure to potential carcinogenic agents in the work environment can also be identified. While some patients will continue in their denial, specific details on smoking and/or alcohol history should be obtained.

Objective evaluation includes a general examination of overall strength, range of motion, and overall functional abilities. This part of the evaluation will need to be adjusted to the patient's tolerance, the strategy being to proceed from the general to the specific.

The pulmonary aspect of the evaluation needs to be as inclusive as possible in order to establish the most appropriate treatment plan and maximize patient progress. Rate and rhythm of breathing are determined by the number of breaths per minute, normal being between 12 and 20. Inspirations should be followed by expirations at a ratio of 1 : 2. A normal breathing pattern is diaphragmatic, with no use of accessory musculature, and has the rate and rhythm described above.[75,76]

In the inspection of the thorax any structural abnormalities such as pectus excavatum, pectus carinatum, kyphosis, and/or scoliosis should be noted. Measurements at the axilla and xiphoid process circumferentially will reveal relative chest mobility with maximal inspiration. Strength of trunk and abdominal musculature, along with specific range of motion, should be noted. Dyspnea, if present, should be graded both at rest and upon activity. Coughing should be assessed for productivity and effectiveness, with a description of the sputum obtained. Since skill level in percussion and auscultation among physical therapists varies, the determination of breath sounds as present, decreased, or absent should serve as the minimal finding, with more specific elaboration if possible.[75,76]

Following the preoperative examination, a physical therapy program is designed to meet the specific needs of each patient. The four areas that should be covered are preoperative patient instruction, immediate postoperative exercise, progressive overall exercise, and instruction in a home exercise program. Preoperative instruction educates the patient as to the importance of postoperative exercise and coughing, specific coughing techniques, diaphragmatic and segmental breathing, lower extremity exercise, and proper body alignment. Immediately following surgery the exercise program will consist of coughing with assistance, diaphragmatic and segmental breathing, and lower extremity exercise. The progressive aspect of the exercise program will emphasize trunk mobility exercises, postural instruction, active lower extremity exercise, and progressive ambulation, ending with home exercise guidelines.

Preoperative Instruction

Preoperative instruction on coughing should emphasize the importance of postoperative coughing, with a demonstration of both the manual assistive and the independent coughing techniques to be followed by a return demonstration by the patient. It should be explained to the patient that coughing helps to keep the lungs and airways clear of secretions and will reduce the risk of pneumonia or further complications after surgery. Independent coughing should be encouraged not only every 30 minutes while awake but also with every change of position. Coughing will be most productive if performed approximately 20 minutes following a change of position.

The best position for an effective cough is with the knees and hips flexed to avoid stressing the abdominal musculature. If the patient is supine, the legs can be flexed, or the patient can sit at the bedside with the legs fixed at the edge. The incision should be supported during coughing to reduce the pain accompanying the cough. As the patient inhales and then coughs, a small pillow or towel roll will support the incision by applying firm pressure directly over the site.

Independent coughing is accomplished as the patient takes three huffs of air, each huff being slightly longer than the previous and the final breath being a deep inspiration. A strong cough can then be produced with the mouth kept open and should be repeated a minimum of five times or until any secretions are expelled.

The purpose of the manual assistive cough is to ensure maximal clearing of the lung and airway secretions by assisting the patient to produce a forceful cough. Since the bed provides a firm surface against which to compress the abdomen, the patient should be positioned supine with hips and knees flexed. The therapist's hands are placed on the abdomen of the patient between the rib cage and the umbilicus. The patient is instructed to take a deep breath and cough on the count of three by the therapist. The therapist says "one, two, three, cough," simultaneously applying a quick downward force to the patient's chest as the patient attempts to cough. This procedure is repeated three to five times, each attempt being slightly stronger according to the patient's tolerance. Patients are generally apprehensive during this procedure and may unknowingly splint to avoid pain. If the patient is relaxed and is reassured in advance that the procedure will begin gently and progress to the patient's tolerance, success will be more likely, enabling the patient to independently produce an earlier effective cough.

Proper breathing techniques are also discussed at the preoperative stage, with instruction in and demonstration of pursed-lip, diaphragmatic, and segmental breathing techniques. The patient is advised that proper breathing will allow air to enter all areas of the lung more completely, will increase the effectiveness of the respiratory muscles, increase chest mobility, decrease pain, and decrease the risk of developing pneumonia.

In pursed-lip breathing the patient is instructed to breathe in through the nose and out through the mouth with the lips pursed as if trying to blow out a candle. The ratio of inspiration to expiration is 2:1, with the emphasis on complete emptying of the lungs. This technique will force the patient to slow down the rate of breathing and is especially useful during periods of pain and overall anxiety.

Diaphragmatic breathing allows the patient to improve the effectiveness of the diaphragm by placing both hands over the upper abdomen while attempting to expand the abdomen by pushing the inhaled air up and against the hands. The patient slowly exhales and repeats the procedure, each time attempting to isolate the diaphragm.

The last breathing technique is segmental breathing, which is similar to diaphragmatic breathing in that both attempt to direct air flow to specific areas. As the name implies, the patient places both hands on the upper, middle, or lower portions of the rib cage during inhalation. An attempt is made to direct the air to the specific portion of the lung under which the hands are placed by pushing the air up and against the hands. Exhalation is again slow and thorough, and this procedure is repeated to include the three segments noted above.

To maintain adequate circulation and prevent the development of thrombophlebitis in the lower extremities, instruction is given in active and isometric exercises for the legs while the patient is confined to bed. These exercises can include ankle pumping, ankle circles, quadriceps setting, hamstring setting, knee flexion, knee extension, gluteal setting, hip abduction, and hip flexion. A selection of three to four of the above exercises that involve the entire extremity is made, and the patient is instructed to repeat each exercise 10 times every waking hour.

Last, the patient is advised concerning the relationship between good posture and proper body alignment with maximal chest mobility. While pain may be a strong influence, splinting toward the site of the incision and its resulting postural deviations should be avoided.

Immediate Postoperative Period

Immediately after surgery patients are reexamined to identify specific problems resulting directly from the surgical procedure. Appropriate short- and long-term goals are established, and a treatment plan is initiated. Even on this first postoperative day patients can and should begin the lower extremity bed exercises that were covered during the preoperative evaluation and instruction.

Progressive Overall Exercise

Once patients are extubated (usually on the second postoperative day), they begin coughing independently as previously instructed, while being reminded of the importance of coughing to avoid further complications. Additionally, coughing with manual assistance may be initially required to produce an effective cough.

Also upon extubation, the postoperative breathing program is initiated; patients perform the pursed-lip, diaphragmatic, and segmental breathing exercises, assisted as necessary by the therapist. While these exercises are usually begun with the patient supine, they should progress to being performed in a sitting and later in a standing position as patient tolerance permits. The patient should be encouraged to attempt the maximal chest expansion possible and if this is significantly restricted by pain, appropriate analgesic measures, including transcutaneous electrical nerve stimulation (TENS), should be considered.

Progressive ambulation is usually initiated on or about the second postoperative day. Patients are instructed not only to maintain correct upright posture while integrating a proper breathing pattern during gait, but also to increase their walking tolerance and overall endurance as they are able. The level of independence during ambulation and/or the need for any assistive devices will dictate the degree of physical therapy involvement in this area.

Finally, patients are instructed in trunk mobility exercises upon removal of the chest tubes, typically around the fourth or fifth postoperative day. Patients are encouraged to be as flexible as possible in all trunk movements and to avoid splinting toward the site of the incision. Patients are instructed in basic exercises to include trunk flexion, trunk extension, trunk lateral flexion, and trunk rotation. If postural deviations are noted at this time, additional corrective exercises may be added to the program.

Home Exercise Program

If the postoperative course is an uncomplicated one, most patients are discharged in approximately 5 days. The physical therapy discharge evaluation will determine what, if any, goals have not been met and in turn what the plan for follow-up should be. Most patients will benefit from a home exercise program that includes their hospital-based program, while some patients may remain limited in chest expansion, trunk mobility, ambulation endurance, and/or pain. These cases may be appropriate for outpatient physical therapy or home health referral as indicated.

REFERENCES

1. Silverberg E, Rubera JA: Cancer statistics. CA 38:5, 1988
2. Office on Smoking and Health: The Health Consequences of Smoking: A report of the Surgeon General. Public Health Service, U.S. Dept of Health and Human Services, Rockville, MD, 1982
3. Fontana RS: Lung cancer and asbestos related pulmonary disease. American College of Chest Physicians: A National Correspondence Course. Chicago, 1981
4. Cohen MH, Matthews MJ: Small cell bronchogenic carcinoma: A distinct clinicopathologic entity. Semin Oncol 5:234, 1978
5. Jett JR, Cortese DA, Fontana RS: Lung cancer: Current concepts and prospects. CA 33:2 Mar/Apr 1983
6. Mountain CF, Carr DT, Anderson WAD: A system for the clinical staging of lung cancer. AJR 120:130, 1974
7. Denoix PF: Enquête permanente dans les centres anticancereux. Bull Inst Natl Hyg 1:70, 1946
8. Mountain CF: A new international staging system for lung cancer. Chest suppl. 89:225s, Apr 1986
9. Ginsberg RJ, Goldberg M, Waters PF: Surgery for non-small cell lung cancer. p. 177. In Wonsiewicz M (ed): Thoracic Oncology. WB Saunders, Philadelphia, 1989
10. Magilligan DJ, Duvernoy C, Malik G, et al: Surgical approach to lung cancer with solitary cerebral metastasis: Twenty-five years' experience. Ann Thorac Surg 42:360, 1986
11. Jensik RJ: The role of segmental resection in lung cancer. Chest, suppl., 89:335s, 1986
12. Kulka F, Forrai I: The segmental and atypical resection of primary lung cancer. Lung Cancer 2:99, 1986
13. Guttman R: Results of radiotherapy in cancer of the lung classified as inoperable at exploratory thoracotomy. Cancer 17:37, 1964
14. Brady LW, Cander L, Evans GC, et al: Carcinoma of the lung: Results of supervoltage radiation therapy. Arch Surg 90:90, 1965
15. Perez CA, Stanley K, Grundy G, et al: Impact of irradiation technique and tumor extent in tumor control and survival of patients with unresectable non-oat cell carcinoma of the lung: Report by the Radiation Therapy Oncology Group. Cancer 50:1091, 1982
16. Committee for Radiation Therapy Studies: Preoperative irradiation of cancer of the lung. Cancer 23:219, 1969

17. Shields TW, Higgins GA, Lawton R, et al: Preoperative x-ray therapy as an adjunct in the treatment of bronchogenic carcinoma. J Thorac Cardiovasc Surg 59:49, 1970
18. Warram J: Preoperative irradiation of cancer of the lung: Final report of a therapeutic trial: A collaborative study. Cancer 36:914, 1975
19. Paulson DL: Carcinomas in the superior pulmonary sulcus. J Thorac Cardiovasc Surg 70:1095, 1975
20. Weisenburger T, Gail M, et al: Effects of postoperative mediastinal radiation on completely resected stage II and stage III epidermoid cancer of the lung. N Engl J Med 315:1377, 1986
21. Kirsch MV, Sloan H: Mediastinal metastases in bronchogenic carcinoma: Influence of postoperative irradiation, cell type and location. Ann Thorac Surg 5:459, 1981
22. Cox JD, Byhardt RW, Komaki R: The role of radiotherapy in squamous, large cell and adenocarcinoma of the lung. Semin Oncol 10:81, 1983
23. Chung CK, Stryker JA, O'Neill M, et al: Evaluation of adjuvant postoperative radiotherapy for lung cancer. Int J Radiat Oncol Biol Phys 8:1877, 1982
24. Choi NC: Reassessment of the role of postoperative radiation therapy in resected lung cancer. Int J Radiat Oncol Biol Phys 8:2015, 1982
25. Slawson RJ, Scott RM: Radiation therapy in bronchogenic carcinoma. Radiology 132:175, 1979
26. Hilaris BS, Nori D, Beattie EJ, et al: Value of perioperative brachytherapy in the management of non-oat cell carcinoma of the lung. Int J Radiat Oncol Biol Phys 9:1161, 1983
27. Hilaris MS, Martini N: The current state of intraoperative interstitial brachytherapy in lung cancer. Int J Radiat Oncol Biol Phys 15:1347, 1988
28. Chute CG, Greenberg ER, Baron J, et al: Presenting conditions of 1539 population-based lung cancer patients by cell type and stay in New Hampshire and Vermont. Cancer 56:2107, 1985
29. Minna JD, Higgins GA, Glatstein EJ: Cancer of the lung. p. 507. In DeVita VT Jr, Hellman S, Rosenberg SA (eds): Cancer: Principles and Practice of Oncology. 2nd Ed. JB Lippincott, Philadelphia, 1985
30. Gralla RJ: Issues and agents in chemotherapy of non-small cell lung cancer. Mediguide Oncol 5:1, 1986
31. Aisner J, Hansen HH: Commentary: Current status of chemotherapy for non-small cell lung cancer. Cancer Treat Rep 65:979, 1981
32. Ruckdeschel JC, Finkelstein DM, Ettinger DS, et al: A randomized trial of the four most active regimens for metastatic non-small cell lung cancer. J Clin Oncol 4:14, 1986
33. Finkelstein DM, Ettinger DS, Ruckdeschel JC: Long term survivors in metastatic non-small cell lung cancer. J Clin Oncol 4:702, 1986
34. Miller TP, Chen T, Coltman CA, et al: Effect of alternating combination chemotherapy on survival of ambulatory patients with metastatic large cell and adenocarcinoma of the lung. J Clin Oncol 4:502, 1986
35. Bitran JD, Golomb HM, Hoffman PC, et al: Protochemotherapy in non-small cell lung carcinoma: An attempt to increase surgical resectability and survival. A preliminary report. Cancer 57:44, 1986
36. Kris MG, Gralla RJ, Casper ES, et al: Complete response with chemotherapy in non-small cell lung cancer (NSCLC): An analysis of patient characteristics; survival and relapse patterns. Proc Am Soc Clin Oncol 2:202, 1983
37. Richards F, Cooper MR, White DR, et al: Advanced epidermoid lung cancer. Prolonged survival after chemotherapy. Cancer 46:34, 1980

38. Livingston RB, Heilbrun LH: Patterns of response and relapse in chemotherapy of extensive squamous carcinoma of lung. Cancer Chemother Pharmacol 1:225, 1978
39. Vosika GJ: Large cell bronchogenic carcinoma—prolonged disease-free survival following chemotherapy. JAMA 241:594, 1979
40. Fram R, Skarin A, Balikian J, et al: Combination chemotherapy followed by radiation therapy in patients with regional stage III unresectable non-small cell lung cancer. Cancer Treat Rep 69:587, 1985
41. Osoba D, Rusthoven JJ, Evans WK, et al: Combined chemotherapy and radiation therapy for non-small cell lung cancer. Semin Oncol 13:121, 1986
42. Cox JD, Samson MK, Herskovic AM, et al: Cisplatin and etoposide before definitive radiation therapy for inoperable squamous carcinoma, adenocarcinoma, and large cell carcinoma of the lung: A phase I-II study of the Radiation Therapy Oncology Group. Cancer Treat Rep 70:1219, 1986
43. Weisenburger TH: Non-small cell lung cancer: Definitive radiotherapy and combined modality therapy. p. 206. In Wonsiewicz M (ed): Thoracic Oncology. WB Saunders, Philadelphia, 1989
44. Takita H, Hollingshead AC, Rizzo DJ, et al: Treatment of inoperable lung carcinoma: A combined modality approach. Ann Thorac Surg 28:363, 1979
45. Trybula M, Taylor SG, Bonomi P, et al: Preoperative simultaneous cisplatin/5-fluorouracil and radiotherapy in clinical stage III, non-small cell bronchogenic carcinoma. Proc Am Soc Clin Oncol 4:182, 1985
46. Martini N, Kris MG, Gralla RJ, et al: The effects of preoperative chemotherapy on the resectability of non-small cell lung carcinoma with mediastinal lymph node metastases (N2M0). Ann Thorac Surg 45:370, 1988
47. Shank B, Sher HI: Controversies in treatment of small cell carcinoma of the lung. Cancer Invest 3:367, 1985
48. Morstyn G. Ihde DC, Lichter AS, et al: Small cell lung cancer 1973-1983: early progress and recent obstacles. Int J Radiat Oncol Biol Phys 10:515, 1984
49. Ihde DC, Makuch RW, Carney DN, et al: Prognostic implications of stage of disease and sites of metastases in patients with small cell carcinoma of the lung treated with intensive combination chemotherapy. Ann Rev Respir Dis 84:481, 1981
50. Zelen M: Keynote address on biostatistics and data retrieval. Cancer Chemother Rep 4(2):31, 1973
51. Hyde L, Wolf J, McCracken S, et al: Natural course of inoperable lung cancer. Chest 64:309, 1973
52. Hansen H: Chemotherapy of small cell carcinoma: A review. Q J Med N Ser 63:275, 1987
53. Matthews MJ, Kanhouwa A, Pickren J, et al: Frequency of residual and metastatic tumors in patients undergoing curative surgical resection for lung cancer. Cancer Chemother Rep 4:63, 1973
54. Fox W, Scadding JG: Medical Research Council comparative trial of surgery and radiotherapy for primary treatment of small celled or oat celled carcinoma of the bronchus: Ten-year follow-up. Lancet 2:63, 1973
55. Salazar OM, Creech RH: "The state of the art" toward defining the role of radiation therapy in the management of small cell bronchogenic carcinoma. Int J Radiat Oncol Biol Phys 6:1103, 1980
56. Greco FA, Richardson RL, Snell JD, et al: Small cell lung cancer: Complete remission and improved survival. Am J Med 66:625, 1979
57. Alberto P, Mermillod B, Joss R, et al: Etopside, cisplatin and doxorubicin in patients with small cell lung cancer: Tumor response and long term survival. Eur J Cancer Clin Oncol 22:701, 1986

58. Feld R, Evans WK, DeBoer G, et al: Combined modality induction therapy without maintenance chemotherapy for small cell carcinoma of the lung. J Clin Oncol 2:294, 1984

59. Catane R, Lichter A, Lee YJ, et al: Small cell lung cancer: Analysis of treatment factors contributing to prolonged survival. Cancer 48:1936, 1981

60. Cohen MH, Creaven PJ, Fossieck BE, et al: Intensive chemotherapy of small cell bronchogenic carcinoma. Cancer Treat Rep 61:349, 1977

61. Seifter EJ, Ihde DC: Therapy of small cell lung cancer: A perspective on two decades of clinical research. Semin Oncol 15(3):278, 1988

62. Ettinger DS, Mehta CR, Abeloff MD, et al: Maintenance chemotherapy versus no maintenance chemotherapy in complete responders following induction chemotherapy in extensive disease small cell lung cancer. Proc Am Soc Clin Oncol 6(689):175, 1987

63. Perez CA, Krauss S, Bartolucci AA, et al: Thoracic and elective brain irradiation with concomitant or delayed multiagent chemotherapy in the treatment of localized small cell carcinoma of the lung: A randomized prospective study by the Southeastern Cancer Study Group. Cancer 47:2407, 1981

64. Seydel HG, Creech R, Pagano M, et al: Combined modality treatment of regional small cell undifferentiated carcinoma of the lung: A cooperative study of the RTOG and ECOG. Int J Radiat Oncol Biol Phys 9:1135, 1983

65. Klastersky J: Therapy of small cell lung cancer: Anything new? Eur J Cancer Clin Oncol 24(2):107, 1988

66. Nugent JL, Bunn PA, Matthews MJ, et al: CNS metastases in small cell bronchogenic carcinoma: Increasing frequency and changing pattern with lengthening survival. Cancer 44:1885, 1979

67. Miller AB, Fox W, Tall R: Five-year follow-up of the Medical Research Council comparative trial of surgery and radiotherapy for the primary treatment of small or oat cell carcinoma of the bronchus. Lancet 2:501, 1969

68. Maassen W, Greschuchna D, Martinez I: The role of surgery in the treatment of small cell carcinoma of the lung. Recent results. Cancer Res 97:107, 1985

69. Maasen W, Greschuchna D: Small cell carcinoma of the lung: To operate or not? Surgical experience in results. Thorac Cardiovasc Surg 34:71, 1985

70. Meyer JA, Comis RL, Ginsberg SJ, et al: The prospect of disease control by surgery combined with chemotherapy in stage I and stage II small cell carcinoma of the lung. Ann Thorac Surg 36:37, 1983

71. Meyer JA, Comis RL, Ginsberg SJ, et al: Phase II trial of extended indications for resection in small cell carcinoma of the lung. J Thorac Cardiovasc Surg 83:12, 1982

72. Shields TW, Higgins GA, Matthews MJ, et al: Surgical resection in the management of small cell carcinoma of the lung. J Thorac Cardiovasc Surg 84:481, 1982

73. Ihde DC: Current status of therapy for small cell carcinoma of the lung. Cancer 54:2722, 1984

74. Murphy M, Samson MM: Physical therapy for the oncology patient. Abby Medical Conference presentation. Los Angeles, 1982

75. Kigin CM: Evaluation and treatment of surgical patients: Chest physical therapy for the postoperative or traumatic injury patient. Phys Ther 61:20, 1981

76. Zadai CC: Evaluation and treatment of the medical patient: Chest physical therapy for the acutely ill medical patient. Phys Ther 61:42, 1981

3 | Rehabilitation of the Head and Neck Cancer Patient

William Lee Roberts

The physical therapist may become involved with the head and neck cancer patient as a result of surgery that may cause shoulder/neck dysfunction. In addition to physical deficits, the physical therapist must be ready to deal with many psychosocial issues related to cosmetic changes resulting from head and neck cancer surgery. This chapter will examine head and neck cancer, beginning with relevant statistics, current staging methodology, and current multimodal antineoplastic treatments. Special emphasis will then be given to physical therapy intervention and the quality of life after treatment.

RELEVANT STATISTICS

Head and neck cancer is one of the easiest cancers to detect. Early symptoms may be noted by the patient and can include color changes in the mouth and tongue, a sore that does not heal in 2 weeks, a lump in the mouth or neck, persistent or unexplained bleeding, numbness in the mouth or lips, persistent dysphagia, or recent onset of nasal obstruction.[1]

Although the functional and cosmetic deficits are very apparent in head and neck cancers, this group of cancers accounts for only 5 percent of all malignancies.[2] It is estimated that there will be 23 new cases per 100,000 males and 8 new cases per 100,000 females in the United States each year. Ironically, almost 32

47

percent of these small numbers of patients diagnosed will eventually die of the disease.[3]

Approximately 80 percent of all head and neck cancers arise from the mucosa of the aerodigestive tract.[2,4,5] Of these, the most common malignant neoplasm of the head and neck is of the squamous cell carcinoma type, which has a favorable prognosis if treated in the early stages (T1 or T2) but a much poorer prognosis in the later stages.[6,7]

The most commonly listed causes of head and neck cancers are tobacco and alcohol abuse.[3] Some authors have suggested that use of alcohol in concert with smoking is among the most common etiologic factors of head and neck cancers.[2,5] When linked together, the risk of cancer is estimated to be 2.5 times as great as for nonsmokers/nondrinkers.[3,8]

Cancers of the upper aerodigestive tract are considered collectively as cancers of the head and neck, including lips, oral cavity, oropharynx, naso-pharynx, hypopharynx, larynx, nose and sinuses, ears, and salivary glands.[8] Of these sites, the most common in descending order of incidence are the larynx, oral cavity, pharynx, and salivary glands.[2,4,5,9,10] Table 3-1 shows the incidence of each type of cancer in the general population. Blitzer attributed the differences noted between white and nonwhite males to a difference in incidence, a difference in success of treatment, or an error in data collection.[3] Some authors have explained the increase in oral and oropharyngeal cancers by the increased use of smokeless tobacco, which has been closely linked with cancer of the cheek and gums.[11] Further, the incidence of head and neck cancer primaries has been shown to increase with age.[3] Nasopharyngeal cancer has often been linked to previous infection with the Epstein-Barr virus, especially among descendants of Chinese from the Canton region.[6,8]

The first outward manifestations of most head and neck cancers are often noticed initially by the primary care physician or dentist in the form of white patches (leukoplakia) and/or red patches (erythroplakia) in the mucosa.[8] In the absence of these patches or other symptoms, unilateral firm lymph nodes in the neck may be the first sign noted by the patient. The physician must carefully evaluate these problems to determine if a diagnosis of cancer is correct. If this diagnosis is established, the treatment of head and neck cancer involves the primary goals of cancer eradication, maintenance of normal function, and acceptable cosmetic appearance.[2,12]

Table 3-1. Mortality per 100,000 Persons, 1970–1979

	White Males	White Females	Nonwhite Males	Nonwhite Females
Oral and oropharynx	4.6 (−3%)[a]	1.5 (+39%)	6.5 (+56%)	1.7 (+30%)
Salivary gland	0.4 (−14%)	0.2 (−21%)	0.3 (0%)	0.2 (21%)
Nasopharynx	0.4 (+13%)	0.2 (+39%)	0.6 (+39%)	0.2 (+88%)
Ear, nose and sinus	0.4 (−32%)	0.2 (−42%)	0.5 (−30%)	0.2 (−19%)
Larynx	2.7 (+5%)	0.4 (+53%)	3.7 (+68%)	0.5 (+54%)

[a] Data in parentheses are percentage change from the 1950s. (Adapted from Blitzer,[3] with permission.)

STAGING

Staging of head and neck cancer follows the TNM (tumor-node-metastasis) system according to guidelines established by the American Joint Committee for Cancer Staging and End Results Reporting (AJC). The primary lesion is denoted as T1, T2, T3, or T4 (Table 3-2). The N denotes metastasis to regional lymph nodes, and the M represents the level of distant metastasis[7] (Tables 3-3 and 3-4). According to current estimates the staging of all head and neck tumors except those of the thyroid have a uniform N classification based on the size, number, and laterality of the affected nodes.[13]

A general physical examination with appropriate scans and radiographs should be performed to assist the physician in properly staging the tumor. One type of procedure, the endoscopic examination, helps to rule out the possibility of a second primary lesion in the respiratory or alimentary tract but should not be used prior to radiologic evaluation, as swelling caused by the endoscopic procedure itself could be incorrectly assessed as a tumor.[7]

In the ideal surgical candidate, a score of 60 or higher on the Karnofsky Performance Scale is often needed for postoperative rehabilitation to be successful.[7] The Karnofsky Performance Scale, which is a performance evaluation tool that allows the physician or allied health professional to anticipate how the patient may recover following surgery/treatment, is based on the patient's current independence and activity level (see Table 3-5).

Some authors have questioned the validity of the TNM system and have proposed alternatives for staging the tumor. In a study by Moore et al., the surface diameter of the cancer was found not to correlate or to correlate in-

Table 3-2. T Categories for Head and Neck Cancer

T	Oral Cavity/ Oropharynx	Nasopharynx	Hypopharynx	Larynx
TX	Tumor cannot be assessed	Tumor cannot be assessed	Tumor cannot be assessed	Tumor cannot be assessed
T0	No primary evidence of disease	No primary evidence of disease	No primary evidence of disease	No primary evidence of disease
TIS	Carcinoma in situ	Carcinoma in situ	Carcinoma in situ	Carcinoma in situ
T1	Tumor less than or equal to 2 cm (dia)	Tumor confined to one site	Tumor confined to site of origin	Tumor confined to site of origin
T2	Tumor greater than 2 cm and less than or equal to 4 cm	Tumor in more than one site	Tumor involving adjacent region or site	Tumor involving adjacent region or site
T3	Tumor greater than 4 cm	Extension beyond region	Extension beyond region	Extension beyond region
T4	Massive tumor with deep invasion	Massive tumor with deep invasion	Massive tumor with deep invasion	Massive tumor with deep invasion

(Adapted from Brady and Davis,[16] with permission.)

Table 3-3. N Categories for Head and
Neck Cancer

N	Clinical Description of Node(s)
NX	Nodes cannot be assessed
N0	No nodes positive
N1	Single homolateral node less than or equal to 3 cm (dia)
N2	Single homolateral node 3 to 6 cm or multiple homolateral nodes greater than 6 cm
N2a	Single positive homolateral node 3 to 6 cm
N2b	Multiple positive homolateral nodes greater than 6 cm
N3	Massive homolateral, contralateral, or bilateral nodes
N3a	Massive homolateral nodes greater than 6 cm
N3b	Massive bilateral nodes
N3c	Massive contralateral nodes only

(Adapted from Brady and Davis,[16] with
permission.)

versely with the aggressiveness of tumors larger than 2 cm. They speculated that
a better predictor may be the thickness of the tumor itself, as has already been
demonstrated in other types of cancer.[14]

Another argument, presented by Ahmad et al.,[15] is that the current staging
system under the AJC guidelines has led to some misinterpretation in that
certain types of tumors with favorable prognoses are classified in the advanced
stages. In their study, patients with T1N0M0 (stage I), T2N0M0 (stage II), and
T1N1M0 (stage III) all had similar survival rates. According to the AJC system,
however, the more advanced stages should have shown a poorer prognosis,
which has led these authors to question the validity of the TNM staging system.[15]

Table 3-4. Stage Groupings

Stage	TNM Groups
I	T1 N0 M0
II	T2 N0 M0
III	T3 N0 M0; any T1 or T2 or T3, N1 M0
IV	T4 N0 M0; any T N2 or N3 M0; any T any N M1

(Adapted from Brady and Davis,[16] with
permission.)

Table 3-5. Karnofsky Performance Scale

100	Normal, no complaints, no evidence of disease
90	Able to carry on normal activity; minor signs or symptoms of disease
80	Normal activity with effort, some signs or symptoms of disease
70	Able to care for self, unable to carry on normal activity or do active work
60	Occasional assistance required, but able to care for most personal needs
50	Considerable assistance and frequent medical care required
40	Disabled, special care and assistance required
30	Severely disabled, hospitalization indicated although death not imminent
20	Very sick, hospitalization necessary, active support treatment necessary
10	Moribund, fatal processes progressing rapidly
0	Dead

(Adapted from Snow,[7] with permission.)

CURRENT MULTIMODAL ANTINEOPLASTIC TREATMENTS

Early diagnosis and treatment often result in high cure rates, with the prognosis depending upon cell type, metastases, and the physical condition of the patient. The patient may complain of certain symptoms during and after treatment. For example, oral cancer can refer pain to the ear, but with early intervention and treatment the chance of a cure is very good.[8] Another example is cancer of the larynx, which when treated by radiation therapy or surgery can result in temporary loss of speech and taste.[16] It is clear from these examples that proper dental care as well as good nutrition (with use of a gastric or nasogastric tube if necessary) must be maintained by the patient during treatment for head and neck cancer in order to allow the physician to properly monitor the effects of the treatment.

Surgery

The physician has three treatment options available—surgery, radiation therapy, and chemotherapy. Results of surgery have been examined by several authors, with particular emphasis on radical and modified neck dissections, to determine the mortality rate from surgery. Attie described results on 313 patients who underwent modified neck dissections, which are often cosmetically superior to and safer than radical neck dissections.[17] Only three of these patients died, all as a result of the disease process. An interesting finding in Attie's study was that even though lymphatic drainage from the thyroid was high and metastatic spread is known to occur early in the disease process, these factors did not affect long-term prognosis.[17] Additionally, Clark et al. argued that a total thyroidectomy may be the best treatment for thyroid cancer even when the possibility of complications is considered. In their study of 160 patients, only 5 patients had complications, 4 of which were classified as short-term deficits.[18] These results are refuted in the literature, with no specific studies citing better treatment protocols.

Two types of reconstructive surgery are commonly practiced following radical neck operations. In the myocutaneous pectoralis major flap procedure, a portion of the chest wall and the pectoralis major muscle along with its blood supply are transposed over surgical wounds in the neck, oral cavity, pharynx, and face to improve function and increase the cosmetic value of surgery.[8] The second procedure involves reconstruction of the mandible and floor of the mouth employing a trapezius osteomyocutaneous flap, which provides well vascularized tissue, and results in a low failure rate even in patients with poor nutritional status or previously irradiated tissue beds.[19]

Some types of head and neck cancers (e.g., squamous cell cancer of the nasal septum and paranasal sinuses and carcinoma of the maxillary sinus) are best treated by both surgery and radiation therapy. As a result of the wide resections often required in these procedures, skin flaps or a prosthetic implant may be necessary to provide adequate speaking and swallowing function.[7]

The only exception found in the literature in which surgery seems to have no role except for biopsy is the treatment of nasopharyngeal cancer. This particular cancer appears to respond more favorably to radiation therapy and/or chemotherapy.[7]

Radiation Therapy

The results of radiation therapy in head and neck cancer treatment have been promising. Radiation therapy is often successful in early lesions, T1 and T2, with cure rates as high as 90 percent; in T3 and T4 lesions with metastases, however, poor results are seen, with cure rates typically as low as 10 percent.[8] In fact, small lesions (T1 and T2) respond very well to radiation therapy alone in most cases. The most common side effect is dehydration of mucous membranes in the upper alimentary tract and a loss of taste, which occasionally lasts for years following the treatment.[16]

A significant finding noted in the literature concerns the use of radiation therapy preoperatively and its effects on healing rates following surgery. Many radiation therapists prefer to irradiate all tumors prior to surgery in an effort to destroy well oxygenated surrounding tissue, which may preclude the possibility of local recurrence.[16] Some authors have reported that local complications involving wound healing are common following surgery when preoperative radiation has been employed.[2,20]

Conversely, the results of a retrospective study by Johnson and Bloomer indicated that patients with prior radiotherapy had no increased incidence of postsurgical wound infections compared with patients with no prior radiotherapy treatments.[21] Thus, no definitive conclusion can be drawn with respect to the effects of preoperative radiation at this time.

Chemotherapy

The results of chemotherapy in the treatment of head and neck cancers appear mixed. Some authors contend that its effectiveness in preventing metastasis of head and neck tumors is as yet unproven, citing such factors as advanced stages of disease and poor nutrition as influencing the results of previous studies.[2,22] Others argue that systemic chemotherapy is the treatment of choice in recurrent and metastatic head and neck cancers.[23]

The four most active chemotherapeutic agents are cisplatin, methotrexate, 5-fluorouracil (5-FU), and bleomycin, with previously reported response rates between 15 and 30 percent. Other commonly used drugs include hydroxyurea, cyclophosphamide, vinblastine, doxorubicin, and various combinations of agents. Major factors to be considered in the selection of chemotherapy combinations are effectiveness, safety, administration, tolerance, and cost.[23]

Multimodal chemotherapy results in higher response rates than single-agent therapy, but drug-induced toxicities are much higher.[23] Tumor regression has been observed in 20 to 40 percent of patients with different combinations of methotrexate, cisplatin, 5-FU, bleomycin, and vinblastine. As a result of the high rate of regression noted with chemotherapy, 50 percent of tumors that are initially unresectable can later be treated surgically or by radiotherapy.[8] In these pilot studies, however, we do not know if cure rates are improved for solid tumors.

The most important prognostic factor in the response of the tumor to chemotherapy appears to be tumor reduction. The greater the reduction, the more positive the prognosis.[23] Local regional failures are the most common reason for distant metastasis in head and neck cancers.[16]

Combined Modalities

Since surgery, radiation therapy, or chemotherapy alone has been unable to cure all head and neck cancers, different combinations of these modalitites have been tried. Historically, chemotherapy alone has not proved effective in treatment of esophageal cancer. Li and Hou in 1987 experimented with a combination of chemotherapy and hyperthermia and reported good response rates but were unable to define the ideal combinations of both.[24]

Sugimachi et al. used radiotherapy with bleomycin and hyperthermia to treat 25 esophageal cancers preoperatively and noted decreases in the size of the tumors. They suggested that surgical resection following this procedure decreased the possibility of metastasis.[25] In yet another study, Arcangeli et al. showed that the immediate response of the tumor and the duration of response were clearly increased by hyperthermia.[26]

The use of hyperthermia and low-dose irradiation in patients with recurrent inoperable malignant tumors resulted in good tumor control for 20 of 23 patients in a 1987 pilot study by Emami and Perez.[27] Further success has been demonstrated in a study by Irish et al. using thermoradiotherapy to treat 18 head and neck cancer patients, in 11 of whom a complete or partial response was achieved. In this study complaints of pain also decreased following the treatment.[28]

Photodynamic Therapy

Another treatment strategy used in head and neck cancer is photodynamic therapy, a modality that uses a hematoporphyrin derivative as a photosensitizing agent, which is absorbed by the tumor. When the tumor is then exposed to certain wavelengths of light, the cancerous cells begin to undergo necrosis. Two theories have been proposed for the mechanism of action in photodynamic therapy. According to the most widely accepted mechanism, energy transfer from the excited sensitizers to oxygen producing singlet oxygen, leads to irreversible oxidation. The other mechanism is based on the suggestion that cell necrosis results from damage to the vasculature of the tumor, although studies of this phenomenon have not been reported.[29] Thomas et al. looked at effects of high-dose laser photoirradiation with lasers on esophageal cancers that had been sensitized with a hematoporphyrin derivative and found a marked response in all tumors. Complications occurred in patients subjected to light power higher than 1.5 W.[30] Further studies of both the response to this treatment and the mechanism of its action are clearly needed.

PHYSICAL THERAPY INTERVENTION

The importance of rehabilitation is critical to the head and neck cancer patient. Cosmetic defects may not initially reflect the underlying problems with muscle alignment and loss of function, and therefore the physical therapist must carefully examine and treat the patient's musculoskeletal deficits in a comprehensive fashion.

The examination should thoroughly cover the following areas:

- Review of prior medical history to correctly identify any previously existing conditions that may affect the surgical outcome (preferably seen preoperatively)
- Visual inspection of the wound, noting color and any edema present

- Assessment of range of motion (both active and passive), with emphasis on the neck and shoulder areas on the affected side
- Evaluation of strength in the affected areas
- Assessment of head mobility in supine, sitting, and standing positions, with any changes noted
- Evaluation of posture, with emphasis on head, neck, and shoulder placement
- Assessment of sensation in the neck and shoulder areas on the affected side

This examination is necessary for all types of head and neck surgery patients in order to identify areas of emphasis for the rehabilitation program. In radical neck dissection the sternocleidomastoid and omohyoid muscles, the spinal accessory nerve, the anterior, external, and internal jugular veins, and the external maxillary artery are excised, along with the lymphatic groups in the anterior and posterior triangles. In comparison, a modified radical neck procedure removes the same muscles and lymphatics and the internal jugular vein but spares the spinal accessory nerve. A functional neck dissection removes only the lymphatics and spares all muscles, nerves, and vessels.[31]

Radical neck dissection can result in serious disability of the shoulder on the operated side due to severance of the spinal accessory nerve. Specific deficits may include a painful shoulder, trapezius muscle paralysis resulting in a rotated scapula, and a loss of range in the shoulder.[32] Loss of trapezius muscle function removes the "passive support" for the shoulder, causing the scapula to rotate medially and deviate laterally. This requires the sternoclavicular joint to bear the weight of the arm, thus contributing to clavicle subluxation.[33] If unsupported, this deficit can result in loss of scapular fixation, where the patient is limited in active motion to approximately 120 to 130 degrees of flexion and 90 degrees of abduction.[34]

Radical neck dissection can decrease range of motion in the head and neck region as a result of the patient guarding against incisional pain.[32] The patient may subsequently develop chronic pain in the affected shoulder, complicated by poor posture and ligamentous strain. In addition, the unopposed action of the pectoralis muscles promote sloping and sagging of the shoulder girdle.[31]

Donovan et al. reviewed the rehabilitation process of the 1960s at M.D. Anderson Cancer Center and found that patients consistently complained of pain and loss of function in light of high compliance with their physical therapy programs. The study found that trapezius dysfunction was a significant factor contributing to these deficits and concluded that future physical therapy intervention should give special attention to trapezius function and rehabilitation.[31]

Herring et al. describe a radical neck syndrome consisting of "constant pain in the shoulder joint, occasional pain in the sternoclavicular joint, decreased ROM [range of motion] during shoulder abduction, and limited motion secondary to skin-flap contraction."[33] The level of severity was variable and was suggested to be due to the concurrent innervation of trapezius by C3 or C4.

The goals of physical therapy of head and neck surgery patients include: increasing range of motion in the neck and shoulder areas to within normal limits; increasing strength in the affected arm and neck areas to the highest level for the patient (usually a level of "good" is attained in the shoulder area); and preventing postural problems by maintaining scapular/shoulder alignment.[31]

Sufficient wound healing should occur in 10 to 14 days to allow the patient to begin the exercise program for the shoulder and neck. Prior to this, however, it is imperative that the patient be cognizant of proper positioning for the affected shoulder and neck areas. While the patient is seated, the shoulder and upper arm should be supported on a pillow or the arm of a chair to prevent further stretching of the trapezius.[32] The start of the exercise program may be delayed in patients with delayed wound healing or fistula formation and those in danger of carotid "blowout." The risk of carotid blowout is critical approximately 2 weeks after surgery and is the result of arterial disease, radiation effects, or removal of the carotid sheath. This is, unfortunately, the time at which most ROM/strengthening exercises are scheduled to begin. The physical therapist must be ready to modify the exercise program to protect the patient during this critical period, as a blow-out of the carotid is potentially fatal.[34]

Additionally, the physical therapist can help by training other muscles to assist with shoulder function. The levator scapulae, through their action as scapular elevators, can be trained to help maintain level shoulders. Patients are instructed to work on this exercise in front of a mirror. The action of scapular retraction can be assumed by the rhomboids, which results in a balanced counterpull to the action of the pectoralis major. The serratus anterior should be strengthened to assist with scapular stabilization during shoulder flexion and abduction. The patient should be cautioned, however, that even with these muscles fully trained, good strength can be expected only in the shoulder and only within a limited range of motion. Unfortunately, no single muscle group can substitute for the complete loss of the trapezius.[34]

A sample home exercise program is displayed in Figure 3-1. This program is provided to all head and neck patients following surgery at the H. Lee Moffitt Cancer Center and Research Institute in Tampa, Florida. The physical therapist evaluates each patient entering this program and modifies the program to accommodate specific patient needs or restrictions.

The physical therapist may be further involved with the head and neck patient if problems with decreased sensation are noted. A thorough sensory evaluation enables the physical therapist to properly educate the patient with regard to deficits that may be harmful. For example, loss of sensation in the ipsilateral neck or arm would require the patient to use the contralateral arm for procedures such as testing the temperature of bath water, removing pots from the oven, etc.

The physical therapist may need to perform an in-depth pulmonary evaluation, especially if the patient has a long history of smoking. Since smoking has been implicated as one of the key factors contributing to head and neck cancer, the possibility of the patient having pulmonary problems, such as chronic obstructive pulmonary disease (COPD), can be well appreciated. The physical therapist must carefully evaluate the severity of dyspnea for the patient and note

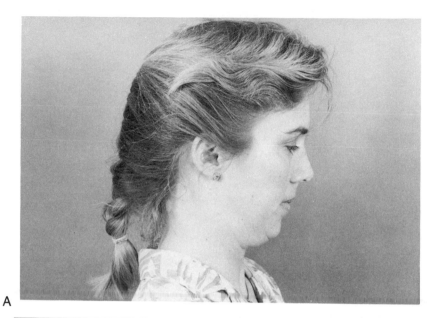

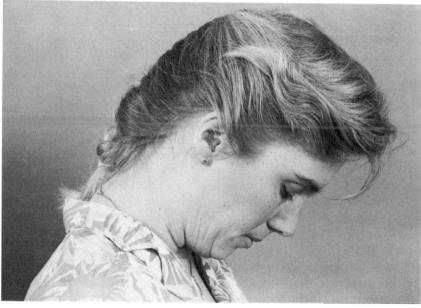

Fig. 3-1. A sample home exercise program. (**A**) Chin tuck. Draw chin back toward the neck while head is held upright (note arrow showing motion). Hold and count to 5. Relax. (**B**) Neck flexion. Place chin on the chest and then return to the upright position. Do not tilt head back! (*Figure continues.*)

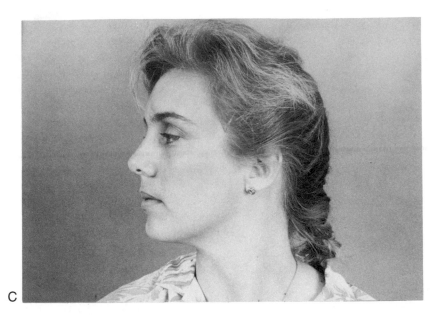

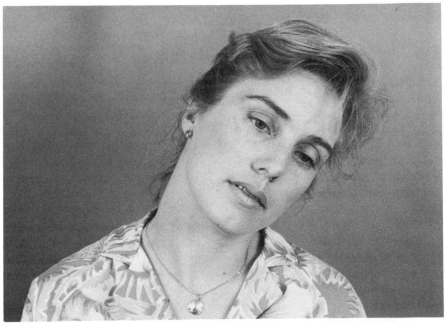

Fig. 3-1. (*Continued*). (**C**) Neck rotation. Keep chin level. Rotate head and look over shoulder, then alternate to the other side (right rotation demonstrated). (**D**) Lateral bending. While looking straight ahead, move left ear towards the left shoulder and then repeat on the right side (left bending demonstrated). Keep shoulders level. (*Figure continues.*)

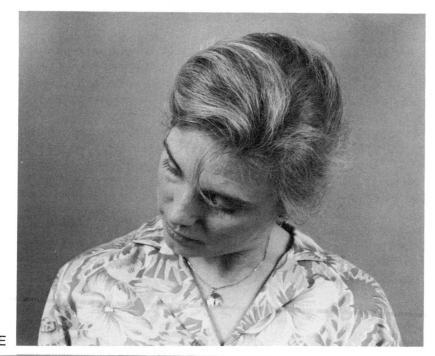

Fig.   3-1. (*Continued*). (**E**) Circumduction. Place chin on chest. Move chin in a smooth arc from shoulder to shoulder (right circumduction demonstrated). (**F**) Pendulum exercise. Stand with body slightly bent forward. Pointing at the floor with the index finger, draw imaginary circles, at first small and then larger. Limit body motion. (*Figure continues.*)

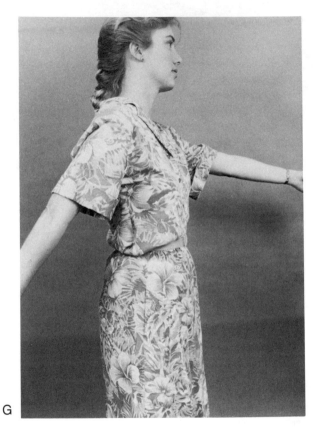

Fig. 3-1. (*Continued*). (**G**) Arm swings. With arms held loosely at sides, swing arms backward and forward in a reciprocal pattern. (*Figure continues.*)

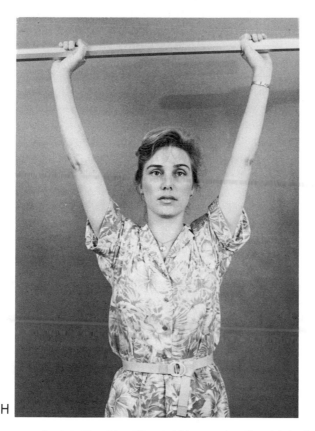

H

Fig. 3-1. (*Continued*). (**H**) Shoulder lift. Hold broom handle with both hands at waist level. While keeping arms straight, raise the broom over the head (demonstrated in highest position). Return to start position. Relax.

any conditions that might increase the breathlessness. Further, the patient's ability to cough and effectively clear secretions will need close attention, as coughing will increase intrathoracic pressure and could promote increased pressure on the carotid artery. The cough itself may be limited by decreased chest or costal excursion as a result of guarding against pain or, as in the case of COPD, as a result of decreased inspiratory efforts. The COPD patient utilizes accessory muscles (e.g., sternocleidomastoid and platysma) to assist with elevation of the rib cage during inspiration. As a result of the sternocleidomastoid being removed in a radical neck dissection, postoperatively the patient may become dyspneic with even mild exertion.

The physical therapist must teach the patient energy conservation procedures as well as breathing exercises to assist the patient with the rehabilitation process. Energy conservation in performing activities of daily living will aid in decreasing dyspnea on exertion. Problems arise for the head and neck patient in the proper positioning (e.g., Trendelenburg) for some breathing exercises, which would promote increased pressure on the neck and the carotid artery. A modified position, such as lying on the side, may be less traumatic and safer for the patient. After the patient is properly positioned, pursed lip breathing exercises should be taught in which the patient breathes in through the nose and out through pursed lips. This procedure creates a back pressure in the lungs, which helps to prevent the airway from collapsing rapidly and thereby controls the amount of air in the lung. There are generally no contraindications to pursed lip breathing, but the physical therapist should monitor the patient closely and discontinue treatment if dyspnea worsens.[34]

The use of physical therapy modalities with the head and neck cancer patient has not been well documented. Heat modalities are generally contraindicated because of decreased sensation in the neck area as well as the vascular concerns noted earlier. Postoperative use of ice packs may be beneficial if edema in the neck and facial areas is a problem but must again be monitored closely because of concerns about decreased sensation.

Luk et al. discussed the importance of a thorough licensing program for hyperthermia operators, which could include physical therapists.[35] This area of physical therapy intervention needs further research to determine the feasibility and appropriateness of physical therapy involvement.

FUNCTIONAL OUTCOME/QUALITY OF LIFE

As mentioned previously, head and neck cancers may result in severe cosmetic problems, which can be disfiguring and can cause a great deal of emotional trauma. Probably the greatest obstacle encountered by the patient is the problem of mastication following major resections.[32] Many patients will note problems with swallowing (dysphagia), particularly if they received preoperative radiation or laryngeal surgery. The physical therapist must be prepared to work with the occupational therapist, speech pathologist, and maxillofacial prosthodontist in the total rehabilitation process, as feeding skills and swallowing are not primary responsibilities of most physical therapists.

Additional problems for head and neck cancer patient can occur as a result of surgery. For example, surgical resection of some tumors of the maxilla often results in functional losses due to significant removal of the hard palate, which make prosthesis fitting difficult if not impossible.[36] An associated problem for the head and neck patient may be pain caused by metastasis, radiation therapy, chemotherapy, ulceration, or the presence of certain irritating substances in the mouth such as food.[32] The occupational therapist may need to be involved with the patient in the fabrication of positioning devices and slings, in training for activities of daily living, and in emphasizing upper extremity function.[37]

Olson and Shedd examined the outcomes for 51 patients following treatment and found that the patients' perceptions of their surgery varied greatly. Of these patients, 28 had undergone a laryngectomy procedure while 23 had other major surgery. Physical appearance scored highest as the area of importance for the nonlaryngectomy group, while speech problems were identified by 92 percent of all patients studied. This study also revealed minor sensory deficits in hearing and vision for certain nonlaryngectomy patients whose surgery involved the seventh, eleventh, and twelfth cranial nerves. All patients were independent in activities of daily living, and coping ability was judged to be good to adequate in 93 percent of them.[38]

In view of these findings, it may be concluded that these patients may need to modify their life-styles by establishing different eating habits, dress appearance, etc. This does not necessarily mean that patients need to change daily social activities; rather they should be encouraged to maintain their previous social contacts. Given the cosmetic deficits noted with head and neck surgery, I have generally noted that the quality of life of these patients is generally improved following an appropriate rehabilitation program.

ACKNOWLEDGMENT

Photographs by Becky Sexton-Larson.

REFERENCES

1. Daly KM: Oral cancer: Everyday concerns. Am J Nurs 79:1415, 1979
2. Rubin P (ed): Clinical Oncology: A Multidisciplinary Approach. 6th Ed. American Cancer Society, Atlanta, 1983
3. Blitzer PH: Epidemiology of head and neck cancer. Semin Oncol 15:2, 1988
4. Batsakis JG: Tumors of the Head and Neck: Clinical and Pathological Considerations. 2nd Ed. Williams & Wilkins, Baltimore, 1979
5. Suen JY, Myers EN: Cancer of the Head and Neck. Churchill Livingstone, New York, 1981
6. Zarbo RJ, Crissman JD: The surgical pathology of head and neck cancer. Semin Oncol 15:10, 1988
7. Snow JB: Surgical management of head and neck cancer. Semin Oncol 15:20, 1988
8. Strong MS, Wang CC, Clark JR: Cancer of the head and neck. p. 132. In Cady, B (ed): Cancer Manual. American Cancer Society, Atlanta, 1986

9. American Cancer Society: Cancer Statistics, 1978. CA 28:17, 1978

10. Del Regato JA, Spjut HJ (eds): Ackerman and del Regato's Cancer, Diagnosis, Treatment, and Prognosis. 5th Ed. CV Mosby, St. Louis, 1977

11. Connolly GN, Winn DM, Hecht SS, et al: The reemergence of smokeless tobacco. N Engl J Med 314:1020, 1986

12. Westbrook KC: Evaluation of patients with head and neck cancer. p. 39. In Neoplasia of Head and Neck. Year Book Medical Publishers, Chicago, 1974

13. Sobin LH, Hermanek P, Hutter RV: TNM classification of malignant tumors: A comparison between the new (1987) and the old editions. Cancer 61:2310, 1988

14. Moore C, Flynn MB, Greenberg RA: Evaluation of size in prognosis of oral cancer. Cancer 58:158, 1985

15. Ahmad K, Kim YH, Fayos JV: Head and neck cancer: Reliability of American Joint Committee's staging system as prognostic indicator. Acta Oncol 26:173, 1987

16. Brady LW, Davis WD: Treatment of head and neck cancer by radiation therapy. Semin Oncol 15:29, 1988

17. Attie JN: Modified neck dissection in treatment of thyroid cancer: A safe procedure. Eur J Cancer Clin Oncol 24:315, 1988

18. Clark OH, Levin K, Zeng Q, et al: Thyroid cancer: The case for total thyroidectomy. Eur J Cancer Clin Oncol 24:305, 1988

19. Dufresne D, Cutting C, Valauri F, et al: Reconstruction of mandibular and floor of mouth defects using the trapezius ostemyocutaneous flap. Plast Reconstr Surg 79:687, 1987

20. Ballantyne AJ: Surgical modifications necessary after radiation therapy in treatment for head and neck cancer. p. 85. In Neoplasia of Head and Neck. Year Book Medical Publishers, Chicago, 1974

21. Johnson JT, Bloomer WD: Effect of prior radiotherapy on postsurgical wound infection. Head Neck Surg 11:132, 1989

22. Glick JH, Taylor SG: Integration of chemotherapy into a combined modality treatment plan for head and neck cancer: A review. Int J Radiat Oncol Biol Phys 7:229, 1981

23. Al-Sarraf M: Head and neck cancer: Chemotherapy concepts. Semin Oncol 15:70, 1988

24. Li D, Hou B: Preliminary report on the treatment of esophageal cancer by intraluminal microwave hyperthermia and chemotherapy. Cancer Treat Rep 71:1013, 1987

25. Sugimachi K, Kai H, Matsufuji H, et al: Histopathological evaluation of hyperthermo-chemo-radiotherapy for carcinoma of the esophagus. J Surg Oncol 32:82, 1986

26. Arcangeli G, Benassi M, Cividalli A, et al: Radiotherapy and hyperthermia: Analysis of clinical results and identification of prognostic variables. Cancer 60:950, 1987

27. Emami B, Perez CA: Combination of surgery, irradiation, and hyperthermia in treatment of recurrences of malignant tumors. Int J Radiat Oncol Biol Phys 13:611, 1987

28. Irish CE, Brown J, Galen WP, et al: Thermoradiotherapy for persistent cancer in previously irradiated fields. Cancer 57:2275, 1986

29. Gluckman JL, Warner M, Shumrick K, et al: Photodynamic therapy: A viable alternative to conventional therapy for early lesions of the upper aerodigestive tract? Arch Otolaryngol Head Neck Surg 112:959, 1986

30. Thomas RJ, Abbott M, Bhathal PS, et al: High-dose photoirradiation of esophageal cancer. Ann Surg 206:193, 1987

31. Donovan E, Scheetz J, Shell B: A physical therapy program for neck dissection patients: The M.D. Anderson Cancer Center approach. Rehabil Oncol 6:6, 1988

32. Dietz JH: Rehabilitation Oncology. John Wiley & Sons, New York, 1981
33. Herring D, King AI, Connelly M: New rehabilitation concepts in management of radical neck dissection syndrome: A clinical report. Phys Ther 67:1095, 1987
34. Catlin PA, Barrett S, Morgan J, et al: Competencies and criteria for the entry level physical therapist. Division of Physical Therapy, Department of Rehabilitation Medicine, Emory University School of Medicine, Atlanta, 1975
35. Luk KH, Drennan T, Anderson K: Potential role of physical therapists in hyperthermia in cancer therapy: The need for further training. Phys Ther 66:340, 1986
36. Jacobs JR, Marunick MT: Surgical considerations in maxillofacial prosthetic rehabilitation of the maxillectomy patient. J Surg Oncol 37:29, 1988
37. Bath T: Occupational therapy intervention with the head and neck cancer patient. Rehabil Oncol 6:13, 1988
38. Olson ML, Shedd DP: Disability and rehabilitation in head and neck cancer patients after treatment. Head Neck Surg 1:52, 1978

4 | Rehabilitation of the Breast Cancer Patient

Joyce L. Adcock

As the physical therapy profession moves toward specialization of services, rehabilitation of the patient with cancer is one of the newest and most promising specialties. It requires innovative management, constant clinical research, and, unfortunately, a too plentiful patient population. Breast cancer patients were among the first cancer patients referred to physical therapists in the early to mid-1970s. As the field of cancer rehabilitation expands, management of breast cancers and their secondary problems remains a challenging and dynamic area of treatment. Physical therapists can provide these patients with improved function, increased comfort, and an acceptable cosmetic effect, resulting in restoration of the patient's self-esteem and body image.

STATISTICS

Although breast cancer is often thought of as a woman's disease, it is important to realize that men also may develop it. Male breast cancer is often missed or diagnosed late because it is rare, and therefore many men are seriously involved by the time of diagnosis.[1] According to the American Cancer Society, as of 1989 breast cancer accounts for an estimated 28 percent of cancers in women and represents the second leading cause of cancer-related deaths in the U.S. (after lung cancer). The incidence of breast cancer in men is less than 1 percent.[2] More specifically, 1 out of 10 women and 1 out of 100 men will develop breast cancer at some time in their lives.[3] Total cases of breast cancer in 1989 are estimated at 142,900, of which 900 will be diagnosed in males, with 43,300 persons, including 300 males, dying of breast cancer.[4]

Although 5 year survival rates for all stages of breast cancer have been slowly increasing (to as high as 75 percent), the mortality rate has remained essentially unchanged since the 1930s (see Fig. 4-1). Even more startling is the fact that cancer is the leading cause of death in women ages 35 to 75 and is second only to heart disease in women 75 and older.[4] In spite of early detection, public education, and improved diagnostic and treatment methods, breast cancer continues to threaten the lives of many Americans.

RISK FACTORS

A number of risk factors predispose a man or woman to develop breast cancer. The significance of recognizing these risk factors is that it aids in identification of and appropriate intervention for those individuals at high risk. The risk factors vary for men and women.

In men common risk factors include: (1) age, (2) hereditary predisposition, (3) history of Klinefelter's syndrome, (4) gynecomastia, and (5) cancer therapy.[3] These statistics may be skewed by a delay in diagnosis, as male breast cancer is not common and therefore may be missed. Although few data regarding familial history are available, sporadic studies in the literature substantiate a predisposition to breast cancer as an inherited trait. It is most interesting that for men at familial risk, the first-degree relatives among whom cancer has occurred are both male and female. Klinefelter's syndrome is an abnormal chromosome pattern in males with complex hormone abnormalities. Studies show these males to be at least 20 times more likely to develop breast cancer than the general population.[5] Males with gynecomastia, an overdevelopment of the mammary glands, have a predisposition to develop breast cancer. Men are also at increased risk of developing breast cancer following treatment for other cancers. In particular, men who have been diagnosed with carcinoma of the prostate and have been treated with estrogen have developed breast cancers. Studies appear controversial in that many men have been diagnosed with metastatic disease to the breast, suggesting minimal influence of this risk factor when compared with others. Radiation exposure may also be a predisposing factor in the development of breast cancer.[3]

In women risk factors are much clearer and are well substantiated in the literature owing to the large population available for study. These factors include (1) family history, (2) age, (3) reproductive history, and (4) other breast diseases.[6] Women who have a first-degree relative (mother or sister) with breast cancer are two to three times more likely to develop breast cancer themselves than the general population. If the first-degree relative has had bilateral breast cancer when premenopausal, the risk increases even more. The incidence of breast cancer increases by as much as 80 percent as a woman enters her forties;[6] it levels off between the ages of 45 and 55 years and then rises gradually as the patient grows older.[2] Therefore, postmenopausal women are at greater risk, the highest incidence of breast cancer per 100,000 occurring in women 75 to 79 years old.[2] If a woman has a long menstrual history—that is, menarche starting at a

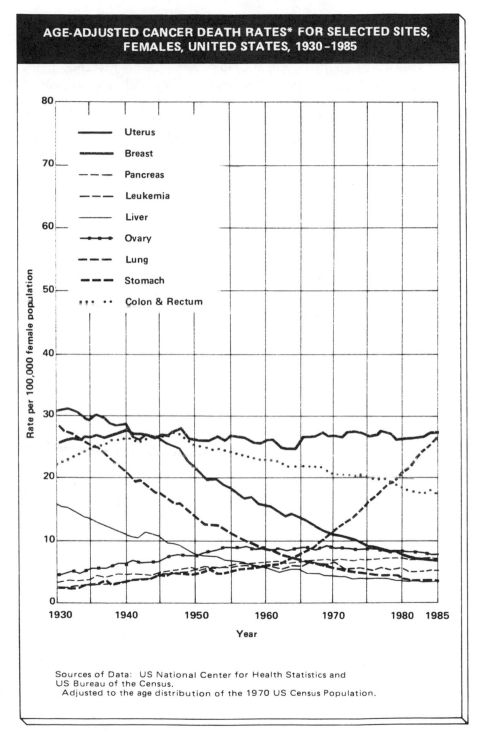

Fig. 4-1. Age-adjusted death rates for selected sites, females, United States, 1930–1985. (From Silverberg and Lubera,[4] with permission.)

young age (before 11 years) and menopause occurring relatively late (after 55 years)—she has a greater risk of developing breast cancer. Women who do not bear children are at even greater risk, and a woman who has her first child before the age of 18 has one-third the risk of a woman who has her first child after age 35. Women who do not nurse their infants have a slightly greater chance of developing breast disease. Cancer can recur in the same breast or the opposite breast. Those women with prior breast cancer are three to four times as likely to develop it again as those with no previous breast disease. The younger the woman is at diagnosis, the greater is her chance of a recurrence. Women with benign breast disease have an increased risk, perhaps four times that of women without such disease, of developing cancer. Some studies show that this increased risk applies only to women with atypical hyperplasia or in those with fibrocystic disease combined with other risk factors.[6,7]

STAGING

Many systems have been developed to stage breast cancer (i.e., to assign the extent of the disease at diagnosis). The historical staging system classified cancers as local, regional, or distant, corresponding, respectively, to disease at the primary site only, spread to the regional lymph nodes, and spread to other areas of the body. Of breast cancers diagnosed from 1979 to 1984, 48 percent were local, 43 percent were regional, and 7 percent were distant.[4]

A more accurate and widely used classification is the American Joint Commission's TNM system, which allows for clinical as well as pathologic staging. Clinical staging is based on the physician's evaluation and noninvasive testing; pathologic staging is based on pathologic evaluation of the tumor, nodes, or other biopsy specimens. This system of classification serves both to identify the extent of tumor and to help define the treatment options.

Figure 4-2 gives a summary of the 1988 TNM classification; T represents the primary tumor, N represents affected regional nodes, and M represents distant metastases. Also noted are the stage groupings. Currently this classification is the most comprehensive and widely accepted staging system.

Staging of breast cancer offers the clinician information related to lymph node involvement, site of tumor, histology of tumor, estrogen receptor assays, and their impact on treatment and prognosis. Those patients with no involvement of axillary lymph nodes have the best chance of complete recovery from their disease. Individuals with one to three positive nodes from a sampling of the axilla also have a favorable prognosis but may require further medical treatment. Those patients with involvement of four or more axillary nodes, supraclavicular nodes, or the internal mammary chain have the gravest prognosis and require aggressive medical intervention.[8] The size of the tumor is also important. Generally, the smaller the tumor the better the prognosis. Tumors less than 2 cm have the most promising prognosis, and if no lymph nodes are involved, 85 percent of patients survive 5 years. The larger the tumor and the greater the extent of regional node involvement, the poorer the survival rate.[6] The type of

Data Form for Cancer Staging

Patient idenification _____

Name _____

Address _____

Hospital or clinic number_____

Age_____ Sex _____ Race_____

Institution identification

Hospital or clinic _____

Address _____

Oncology Record

Anatomic site of cancer _____

Histologic type _____

Grade(G) _____

Date of classification _____

Chronology of classification
(use separate form for each time staged)
[ ] Clinical (use all data prior to first treatment)
[ ] Pathologic (if definitively resected specimen available)

Definitions

Primary Tumor (T)

[ ] TX Primary tumor cannot be assessed

[ ] TO No evidence of primary tumor

[ ] Tis Carcinoma *in situ* ; Intraductal carcinoma, lobular carcinoma *in situ*, or Paget's disease of the nipple with no tumor.

[ ] T1 Tumor 2 cm or less in greatest dimension

[ ] T1a 0.5 cm or less in greatest dimension

[ ] T1b More than 0.5 cm but not more than 1 cm in greatest dimension

[ ] T1c More than 1 cm but not more than 2 cm in greatest dimension

[ ] T2 Tumor more than 2 cm but not more than 5 cm in greatest dimension

[ ] T3 Tumor more than 5 cm in greatest dimension

[ ] T4 Tumor of any size with direct extension to chest wall or skin

[ ] T4a Extension to chest wall

[ ] T4b Edema (including peau d'orange) or ulceration of the skin of breast or satellite skin nodules confined to same breast

[ ] T4c Both T4a and T4b

[ ] T4d Inflammatory carcinoma

Lymph Node (N)

[ ] NX Regional lymph nodes cannot be assessed

[ ] N0 No regional lymph node metastasis

[ ] N1 Metastasis to movable ipsilateral axillary lymph node(s)

[ ] N2 Metastasis to ipsilateral axillary lymph node(s) fixed to one another or to other structures

[ ] N3 Metastasis to ipsilateral internal mammary lymph node(s)

Pathologic Classification (pN)

[ ] NX Regional lymph nodes cannot be assessed

[ ] pN0 No regional lymph node metastasis

[ ] pN1 Metastasis to movable ipsilateral axillary lymph node(s)

[ ] pN1a Only micrometastasis (none larger than 0.2 cm)

[ ] pN1b Metastasis to lymph nodes, any larger than 0.2 cm

[ ] pN1bi Metastasis in 1 to 3 lymph nodes, any more than 0.2 cm and all less than 2 cm in greatest dimension

[ ] pN1bii Metastasis to 4 or more lymph nodes, any more than 0.2 cm and all less than greatest dimension

[ ] pN1biii Extension of tumor beyond the capsule of a lymph node metastasis less than 2 cm in greatest dimension

[ ] pN1biv Metastasis to a lymph node 2 cm or more in greatest dimension

[ ] pN2 Metastasis to ipsilateral axillary lymph nodes that are fixed to one another or to other structures

[ ] pN3 Metastasis to ipsilateral internal mammary lymph node(s)

Distant Metastasis (M)

[ ] MX Presence of distant metastasis cannot be assesssed

[ ] M0 No distant metastasis

[ ] M1 Distant metastasis (includes metastasis to ipsilateral supraclavicular lymph nodes)

Stage Grouping			
[ ] 0	Tis	N0	M0
[ ] I	T1	N0	M0
[ ] IIA	T0	N1	M0
	T1	N1*	M0
	T2	N0	M0
[ ] IIB	T2	N1	M0
	T3	N0	M0
[ ] IIIA	T0	N2	M0
	T1	N2	M0
	T2	N2	M0
	T3	N1	M0
	T3	N2	M0
[ ] IIIB	T4	Any N	M0
	Any T	N0	M0
[ ] IV	Any T	Any N	M1

Note: The prognosis of patients with pN1a is similiar to that of patients with pN0.

Histopathologic Grade (G)

[ ] GX Grade cannot be assessed

[ ] G1 Well differentiated

[ ] G2 Moderately well differentiated

[ ] G3 Poorly differentiated

[ ] G4 Undifferentiated

Staged by _____ M.D.

_____ Registrar

Date _____

Fig. 4-2. Data form for staging of breast cancer. (From American Joint Committee on Cancer Staging—1988: Manual for Staging of Cancer. JB Lippincott, Philadelphia, 1988, with permission.)

breast cancer diagnosed also is related to outcome. Infiltrating ductal carcinoma accounts for 80 percent of all cancers diagnosed, infiltrating lobular carcinoma for 9 percent, and medullary carcinoma for 4 percent. Ductal and lobular carcinomas tend to involve lymph nodes and therefore have a poorer prognosis than those less common tumors that tend not to involve lymph nodes.[9] Some tumors are receptive to estrogen (ER+); patients with such tumors are more likely to respond to hormonal therapy and also tend to be disease-free for longer periods than those whose tumors are estrogen receptor-negative (ER−).[10]

MULTIMODAL ANTINEOPLASTIC TREATMENT

The goals of medical management of breast cancer include (1) preserving life, (2) minimizing the chance of recurrence, and (3) providing the best cosmetic result. The most appropriate treatment of breast cancer remains a controversial issue. Recently the trend has been to minimize surgical intervention and combine other treatment modalities. Common medical treatment includes surgery, radiation, chemotherapy, hormonal therapy, and/or any of these in combination.

Surgical Treatment

The Halsted radical mastectomy was developed in the late 1800s and widely used into the 1950s and 1960s. It involved removal of the skin, the breast, the pectoralis major and minor muscles, and the axillary lymph nodes.[11] In the mid-1900s some surgeons advocated the extended radical mastectomy, which included removal of all the above structures as well as the internal mammary chain, the rib, and the supraclavicular lymph nodes.[12] Both of these procedures left the individual with severe cosmetic and functional deficits.

More recently the surgical intervention most frequently practiced and advocated is the modified radical mastectomy. In this procedure the skin, breast tissue, and a sampling of the axillary nodes are removed. This procedure has been widely accepted and has resulted in a good prognosis. Also, the patients are spared the extreme functional and cosmetic deficits noted with the more radical procedures.[13]

Currently, many surgeons are advocating even less radical procedures. Some of these are: (1) simple, or total mastectomy, in which only the breast is removed and a separate procedure is used to sample the axillary nodes; (2) partial mastectomy, in which the surgeon removes the tumor and a wedge of surrounding breast tissue following B7 radiation treatment; and (3) local wide excision, also called a lumpectomy or tylectomy, followed by radiation treatment. Often axillary nodes are removed separately as in partial mastectomy or in local wide excision.[2]

Radiation Therapy

Radiation treatment is frequently used in the treatment of breast cancers. It is utilized preoperatively for operable tumors, postoperatively with radical and with more conservative surgeries, as a primary treatment for inoperable breast cancers, and as a modality to decrease pain and enhance tissue healing.[14]

Presurgical radiation can be used on operable tumors although this is done infrequently. Its primary effect is to shrink the tumor to a more readily operable size. This approach is most frequently seen in the management of head and neck cancer to substantially reduce the functional and cosmetic deficits. Its application in breast cancer management is not well substantiated in the literature. Many physicians feel that it delays and/or inhibits the effect of necessary surgery.[15]

Postoperative radiation is now a widely accepted procedure, particularly with those patients who elect to have less radical surgical intervention. Its purpose is to destroy any remaining tumor cells following surgery. Initial studies have demonstrated 10-year results comparable with those obtained in patients undergoing the more conventional modified radical mastectomy. These studies began in 1971, with 5- and 10-year survival rates reported in 1977 and 1985.[15] Average radiation dose varies from 4,000 to 5,000 rads to the breast, chest wall, and nodes. This option has become one of the more widely accepted procedures, and women are choosing it in order to maintain an acceptable cosmetic end result.

Radiation has been used as a primary treatment for breast cancer when the patient has refused surgery. Although it has been shown to be helpful, it has not produced a significant "cure rate." It is, however, an excellent modality for some inoperable cancers, particularly in conjunction with chemotherapy. It is often the treatment of choice for advanced breast disease because of its ability to shrink tumor, provide local tissue healing, and decrease pain.[16]

Another form of radiation therapy, practiced since the 1930s, consists of interstitial implants, which remain in the breast for 50 to 60 hours and provide about 2,000 rads of localized treatment. They are usually used in conjunction with excisional biopsy for local regional control. Results obtained with this procedure have been favorable.[2]

Chemotherapy

Chemotherapy is instituted primarily when a patient has regional or distant metastasis. Drugs often used include: (1) alkylating agents, which inhibit cell growth by damaging DNA; (2) antimetabolites, which act in cell mitosis by interfering with the synthesis of DNA and RNA; (3) antibiotics, which adhere to the DNA, inhibiting DNA replication and transcription; and (4) mitotic inhibitors, which prevent mitosis (i.e., cell division).

Treatment of breast cancers began with a single-agent approach, and although 5-year survival rates were promising, 10-year rates did not yield a significant positive effect. With the introduction of multiple agents, survival rates were increased. This resulted in adjustments to combinations, dosage, and frequency of treatment. Although combined agents have shown good effect, no one combination has proved superior to the others. Premenopausal patients with positive lymph nodes show a greater response to treatment than postmenopausal women with positive nodes.[16]

Hormonal Therapy

One of the newest approaches to treatment of breast cancers is hormonal therapy. Hormonal treatment or endocrine manipulation has shown to be effective both in managing metastatic disease and as an adjuvant to primary treatment. Hormonal therapy is referred to as *additive* (adding male or female hormones) or *ablative* (obliterating or removing those organs that produce hormones). As mentioned earlier, hormone receptor assays can be done to determine if a patient is estrogen receptor-positive, in which case she responds to hormonal management. Approximately 50 percent of women are estrogen receptor-positive.[7]

Additive therapies consist of the use of androgens, estrogens, progesterone, and corticosteroids and are widely accepted owing to decreased risk factors as compared with surgical intervention and decreased toxicity responses of some chemotherapeutic agents. Tamoxifen, an antiestrogen, has been one of the most promising and effective modalities for treating breast cancer in postmenopausal women. It is likely that further studies of techniques for manipulation of hormones will be made the next decade of cancer medicine.

Ablative techniques involving x-rays or surgery are not widely used today. Historically it was not uncommon, particularly in premenopausal women, to perform a bilateral oophorectomy. Other surgical interventions include hypophysectomy or adrenalectomy. Obliterating the ovaries, adrenal, or pituitary gland markedly affects hormone production.

PHYSICAL THERAPY INTERVENTION

Both men and women can present with functional and cosmetic deficits that can be reduced or alleviated by physical therapy. Some of these deficits are directly related to their cancers, and others result from prior medical treatment. These deficits include decreased upper extremity mobility, skin breakdown, neuropathic changes, postural changes, and secondary edema. Many of the physical therapy interventions for these problems are not unique and have been developed to manage other pathologies. Some, however, are specific but can be directed toward managing other, non-cancer-related pathologies.

General Considerations

Ideally the therapist's role starts with a pretreatment evaluation of the patient, which allows the therapist and patient to develop a rapport. A brief cognitive and social assessment and an explanation of the physical therapist's role and the intervention provide an opportunity for patients to explore concerns and ask questions that remain confusing to them. The therapist conducts a general functional assessment, which includes mobility, strength, general health, and orientation. This examination would include palpation of nodes;

specific range of motion of neck, shoulder girdle, and upper extremities; hand dominance; skin color; condition of chest wall, upper extremity and clavicular area; fine and gross motor skills; sensation; and bilateral circumferential measurements. The therapist also has the opportunity to begin instruction in postoperative positioning and mobility if surgery is the treatment of choice.

Since the majority of breast cancers do require some type of surgical intervention, the physical therapist plays a critical role in the area of preventive medicine. Therapists have the opportunity to provide treatment as well as to educate patients. If patients understand that early intervention may prevent further problems and complications, they may be more compliant and actively participate in their care.

After surgery the patient may be confined to bed for a day. If so, the arm on the affected side must be sightly abducted and flexed at the shoulder and the

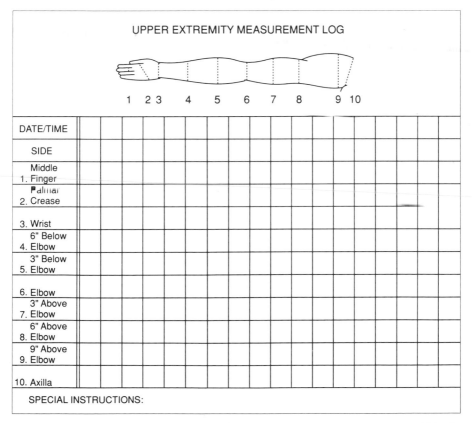

Fig. 4-3. Upper extremity measuring sheet. (Courtesy of Jenkintown Rehabilitation Services, Jenkintown, PA.)

distal aspect of the extremity elevated and supported. This position will inhibit postsurgical edema and avoid protective splinting. If the patient is sitting up on the first day, this posture should also be adopted, with the arm resting on a tray or elevated by using an IV pole sling, as will be discussed later. Postsurgically, circumferential measurements should be taken of the arm to monitor changes in girth (see Fig. 4-3). The patient should be encouraged to actively move the hand, wrist, forearm, and elbow. The rehabilitation nurse or therapist can gently start passive and active-assisted range-of-motion exercises for the shoulder and active-assisted exercises in the supine position. These personnel must be cognizant of the type and extent of the surgical procedure in order not to traumatize the incision or jeopardize healing.

By day 3 many patients are up and about but tend to hold the affected arm against the body with the elbow flexed at 90 degrees, often supporting it with the unaffected arm. This pattern can be detrimental if allowed to persist. Every patient must be encouraged to adopt a more normal posture. By day 4 or 5 patients can be started on an active shoulder exercise program, including active neck range-of-motion exercises, shoulder shrugs, protraction and retraction, active rotation, flexion, and abduction to tolerance. The patient may need to use the opposite extremity to assist with shoulder range of motion. Resistive exercises for the hand, wrist, and forearm also can begin at this time. It is not unusual for patients to experience some pain. They must be reassured that this is to be expected and encouraged to work through it. Generally use of physical therapy modalities is not indicated at this time. As patients improve they should be taught to monitor circumferential measurements, be instructed in the warning signs of infection (see Fig. 4-4), and be given a written program of exercise and a list of hand and arm care (Fig. 4-5). Following discharge patients should return for follow-up assessment to be sure all is stable and that they clearly understand

---

CALL YOUR DOCTOR OR THERAPIST IF THERE ARE CHANGES IN YOUR ARMS

COLOR – redness, streaking or blotching

TEXTURE – arm is softer, harder, skin is rough or indented

TEMPERATURE – arm feels warmer than the other extremity

SIZE – arm feels full or heavy
    – clothing and jewelry do not fit as well
    – increased circumferal measurements of 2/8"
      for more than 3 consecutive days

Fig. 4-4. Patient form listing signs of infection. (Courtesy of Jenkintown Rehabilitation Services, Jenkintown, PA.)

their program. Many patients will have an uneventful course and not require additional physical therapy intervention once they have achieved full mobility and strength.

The majority of breast cancer patients who require physical therapy are seen because of a problem that develops some time after initial medical treatment. At times it seems physical therapy referral may be delayed because these patients may be keeping other medical appointments and receiving radiation and/or chemotherapy. Their condition may not warrant the additional stresses of physical therapy unless this is absolutely necessary.

Treatment of Decreased Mobility

One common, easily correctable problem developed by breast cancer patients is decreased mobility of the upper extremity, particularly at the shoulder girdle. This deficit is most often the result of disuse but is further complicated by superficial and deep soft tissue changes. Prior to initiating any physical therapy program a radiograph should be taken to ensure the integrity of the joint and the absence of metastatic disease in the humerus or related structures. One must examine the chest wall and the axilla carefully to determine if there are adhesions, particularly postsurgically, or disease that may be restricting motion. Patients may also have fibrotic skin changes that inhibit motion, especially if they have received radiation treatment.

Prior to initiating a passive or active exercise program, it is necessary to make sure that the tissue is supple. One of the most effective means of accomplishing this is through deep tissue friction massage using steroid in a petroleum base. This type of massage breaks down adhesions, increases circulation, and conditions the skin. If the patient has completed a course of radiation, hot or cold modalities can be used in conjunction with the massage. Gentle stretching and range-of-motion exercises can follow these modalities to allow for mobility superficially and within the joint capsule itself. If the bones are "healthy," gentle mobilization can be a very effective complement to this treatment approach. As the patient achieves increased passive range, active exercise and functional activities should be encouraged.

Treatment of Skin Problems

Tissue massage, as described above, will enhance the integrity of the skin. Those patients who have wounds caused by delayed healing due to radiation therapy, ulcerated chest walls due to advanced disease, erythemas, or moist exfoliations will require instructions in skin care. Also, a large number of patients may develop herpes zoster on the affected side. General skin care instructions include cleansing the skin with tepid water and no soap, patting the area dry, wearing loose, nonbinding clothing, discontinuing use of skin creams

INFORMATION FOR BREAST CANCER PATIENTS
SPECIAL INSTRUCTIONS FOR HAND AND ARM CARE

1. AVOID CUTS, SCRATCHES, AND IRRITATION
   - use cuticle cream instead of scissors
   - wear heavy gloves and long sleeves when gardening and avoid thorns
   - use rubber gloves for washing dishes and cleaning

2. DO NOT HAVE INJECTIONS OR VACCINATIONS IN THE AFFECTED ARM – ASK TO HAVE THEM ON THE OTHER SIDE

3. AVOID WASPS, BEES, AND OTHER INSECTS
   - call the doctor if you get a wasp or bee sting
   - use insect repellant if you are going to be exposed to insects

4. AVOID BURNS
   - if you smoke, hold your cigarette in the other hand
   - always use a padded glove when reaching into the oven
   - avoid sunburn – use protective sun lotion and tan gradually –
     if possible, cover your affected arm when in the sun (with
     long sleeves or a towel)

5. AVOID BINDING OR SQUEEZING YOUR ARM
   - do not have blood pressure taken in the affected side
   - wear loose jewelry (wrist watch, bracelets, and rings)
   - wear loose sleeves
   - do not carry your handbag on the affected shoulder or in
     the affected hand – carry it on the other side

6. AVOID UNDERARM IRRITATION
   - talk to your doctor and/or therapist before shaving your
     underarm
   - ask your doctor's and/or therapist's advice about deodorant –
     do not use any product which causes a rash or other irritation

7. AVOID STRAINING YOUR ARM
   - let others carry heavy objects
   - do not move furniture
   - ask your therapist's advice about strenuous activities you want
     to do

8. TAKE EXTRA CARE OF YOUR HAND AND ARM
   - use lanolin cream on your hand and arm several times a day
   - in case of minor breaks in the skin (insect bites or scrapes),
     wash the affected area and cover it with a bandage
   - burns or cuts should be seen immediately by a doctor and/or
     a therapist; an antibiotic is usually needed
   - call your doctor or therapist promptly if any sign of infection
     occurs, such as:

       - increased warmth in the affected arm
       - red streaks or reddened areas in the affected area
       - sudden increase in swelling of the affected arm

Fig. 4-5. Hand and arm care instruction sheet. (Courtesy of Jenkintown Rehabilitation Services, Jenkintown, PA.)

or lotions, and avoiding direct exposure to the sun. If the patient develops skin breakdown, healing the tissue and increasing patient comfort become the primary objectives. If the patient has moist desquamation, application of corn starch and topical steroids is helpful. Those patients who have extensive skin breakdown or advanced disease may benefit from cleansing of the area followed by moist to dry dressing using water and hydrogen peroxide or saline solution. Analgesics may decrease some of their discomfort. Patients with herpes benefit from medication primarily. Cool compresses and steroid cream may make them more comfortable and promote healing of the lesions.

Treatment of Neuropathic and Postural Changes

Breast cancer patients can experience neuropathic changes in the upper extremity, including pain, hyperesthesia, paresthesias, weakness, and trophic changes. These problems can stem from tumor infiltration, profound axillary node involvement, radiation-induced injury, surgical insult, or edema. Nerve tissue can be permanently damaged by surgical trauma or advancing disease. Transient entrapments can occur as a result of fibrosis and/or edema; these can be reduced by increased mobility, release of adhesions, and decrease in edema.

It is not uncommon for postsurgical patients to experience short-term superficial sensory loss and radiating pain, which is usually described as aching in quality and which travels distally along the medial upper arm. It usually subsides spontaneously over time (6 months to 1 year). Patients who have entrapment signs and symptoms should receive early treatment to eliminate the cause of the compression and thereby alleviate the symptoms. Those individuals with persistent, long-term neuropathic changes can experience severe disability, which renders the arm dysfunctional. For these patients the therapist must employ protective mechanisms, including instruction in skin care, use of a sling to protect the extremity and enhance balance, and dynamic or static splinting to maintain position and function of the wrist and hand. These patients will also benefit from instruction in the use of adaptive equipment and items that can be operated single-handed if the arm becomes dysfunctional.

Mastectomy patients, particularly those with more radical procedures, tend to develop asymmetrical postures over time. Early intervention emphasizing postural education can serve to inhibit some of these secondary changes. The therapist should note shoulder symmetry on the involved side. At times the shoulder is held in a depressed, protracted position, which often can result in slight lateral flexion and rotation of the neck toward the affected side. Posteriorly one might note the scapula to be markedly abducted, which inhibits normal movement patterns of the shoulder girdle. Simple intervention such as chest expansion exercises, scapular adduction, and shoulder elevation and retraction all help to prevent or decrease these postural changes.

Treatment of Edema

The incidence of secondary arm edema has been decreasing with the advent of less radical surgical intervention. It remains, however, a troubling problem for many patients. These individuals are dependent on the skill and expertise of the therapist as well as on those of the physician. A variety of studies have shown that 6.7 to 62.5 percent of individuals with breast cancer will develop secondary edema in the upper extremity.[17] My past personal experience suggests that this problem is seen in 30 to 40 percent of women. Secondary arm edema may also be seen in 60 to 70 percent of men with breast cancer, usually owing to more severe involvement. In spite of these figures, many physicians and patients alike apparently believe this edema to be an irresolvable problem.

There are a number of contributory causes to the development of edema. Surgery itself may be the primary cause; extensive dissection of the axillary nodes can incapacitate the lymphatic system. Lymph tissues serve as part of the body's immune defense system and the greater the number of nodes dissected, the greater the functional impairment of the lymphatic system. This creates a twofold problem: loss of nodes to circulate lymph fluid and decreased ability to fight infection. Without careful attention to the tissue during surgery, the operation can result in excessive scarring, which promotes adhesions and thereby effectively closes down lymphatic channels. The disease itself can become a contributory cause. Should the tissue be invaded by metastatic disease, this process can literally dam the lymphatic system, prohibiting exchange of fluids. Radiation treatment, used independently or in conjunction with other treatment, can be a significant contributor to edema. Radiation-induced fibrotic tissue becomes thickened and invasive, shutting down the lymphatic channels and rendering the nodes nonfunctional.

Perhaps the most significant and most frequent cause of edema is infection. The main function of the lymphatic system is to remove waste excreted from body tissue. The fluid that it carries contains phagocytes, which digest bacteria, and lymphocytes, which trap and destroy invading cells. If the immune system is compromised, those vital functions do not occur, which makes the extremity susceptible to infection. It is important to point out that patients are vulnerable to *any* type of infection. Systemic infection can precipitate upper extremity edema; the patient does not have to sustain direct trauma to the extremity. Past experience indicates that spontaneous edema (i.e., edema without an identifiable cause) is extremely rare.

Edema is simply an accumulation of excess fluid in the interstitial space. It can be classified into two distinct types: lymphatic edema, in which plasma proteins in the tissues stagnate owing to mechanical insufficiency of lymph drainage, and venous edema, which results in increased capillary pressure and venous obstruction. When the lymphatic system is incompetent, obstructed, or surgically obliterated, proteins and their products accumulate in the tissue space. Edema occurs when there is an imbalance of the affected pressures across the capillary membrane or when there is obstruction to the venous or lymphatic flow. Thus, the tissue has abnormally large quantities of fluid in the intercellular spaces. If this process remains unchecked, collagen tissue tends to be deposited in this protein-rich fluid, eventually leading to fibrosis.

Signs of edema include: (1) marked fullness in the arm due to increased interstitial fluid; (2) color changes, usually reddening; (3) changes in skin temperature; and (4) changes in turgor.

The primary objective of edema management is to treat it before it becomes a long-standing problem. The earlier one intervenes, the quicker and more successful the treatment. In evaluating the edema one must check for signs of infection (see Fig. 4-4), which include redness or streaking of the skin, an increase or decrease in skin temperature, opened or oozing areas, and hard turgor. I advocate the use of an electric skin thermometer. Naturally, the skin temperature will decrease as one moves distally down the extremity. One must compare the affected and unaffected extremity. A decrease or increase in temperature can be indicative of a deep or superficial infection, respectively. Infection demands treatment with a broad-spectrum antibiotic and no aggressive physical therapy initially. Circumferential measurements of both upper extremities should be taken and recorded (Fig. 4-3). This procedure should be repeated by the same person at the same time of day, with the same tape used for each measurement. Circumferential measurements are more expedient than volumetric measurements and allow one to identify localization of edema. Routine range-of-motion tests, a manual muscle test, and sensory evaluation of the neck, shoulder girdle, and upper extremity are indicated. Color, texture, skin condition and temperature must be noted on physical examination. Pretreatment and post-treatment photographs are desirable but not necessary.

As I have gained experience with management of edema, it has become apparent to me that individual patients require their individual protocols. There is no single way to treat this problem. Massage, exercise, elevation, and compression can be used independently or in conjunction with one another. Retrograde massage with a good skin conditioner has been shown to provide transient relief for patients with edema. This technique mobilizes fluid, enhances the health of superficial tissue, and inhibits the laying down of collagen. Unfortunately, in spite of these benefits it does not provide significant long-term relief.

Recently, therapists in the United States have been using manual lymph drainage based on the principles of Emil Vodder. These are specific massage-like techniques designed to displace fluids, thus promoting increased venous return. Those therapists schooled in the Vodder technique have reported positive and rapid results. Manual lymph drainage is reported to have an effect on the autonomic nervous system, reflex pathways, immune system, and smooth muscle.[18] Although not a well established procedure in the United States, it does warrant further study.

Exercise is beneficial to the patient not only to maintain mobility and strength but also to assist in decreasing edema. Isometric upper extremity exercise with elevation uses the natural muscle pump to exert pressure on the vessels that assist in fluid return. It is helpful to use a hand-held T-foam block because once this block is compressed, the patient maintains the contraction and in effect performs an isometric exercise. The patient is instructed not to resume exercise until the T-foam returns to its original shape; this provides a controlled pace, which the patient cannot exceed.

Elevation of the extremity is always helpful. Gravity assists in facilitating normal venous and lymphatic flow. Patients should be encouraged to elevate the affected arm when at rest, both sitting and supine. They should be discouraged from keeping the arm in a dependent position when up and about and encouraged to maintain mobility. Prefabricated foam elevating devices, an inverted quad board, or a towel with webbing suspended from an IV pole can be used to maintain comfortable elevation.

Compression of the edematous extremity is one of the most effective techniques if a patient is an appropriate candidate. Examples of compression therapy range from the mildest application of elastic stockinette to an aggressive pneumatic compression program to serial sleeving.

Single or multiple layers of elastic stockinette provide a quick and easy method to provide constant external compression. Because it is soft and comes in different sizes, it is easily fitted and comfortable to a patient with a painful arm whose skin is in poor condition. It can also be used to assess patients' tolerance for compression or to evaluate whether they are candidates for more aggressive intervention. It is often considered as a primary treatment for those with advanced disease and severe involvement who need to protect the tissue. Elastic stockinette also serves as an interim means to help maintain reduction achieved with pumping. It is relatively inexpensive and disposable, which makes it an excellent choice for those patients with weeping excoriated areas.

Mechanical pumping to achieve edema reduction can utilize a sequential or a single-chamber appliance. The therapist has the choice of selecting a pump that provides pneumatic compression or an appliance that fills with cold water. Because of the diversity of equipment on the market, I recommend the following guidelines when selecting the most appropriate compression unit: the appliance should be washable to ensure that cross-infection between patients does not occur; the pump should have separate timers for inflation and deflation; and it should be possible to independently set pressures for inflation and deflation, so that the patient can receive static compression with a superimposed intermittent component prohibiting refilling of the extremity. Some patients will tolerate use of a cold water pump better than use of a more conventional pneumatic pump. A cold water pump is especially effective when treating a patient who has edema as a result of a resolving infection.

I recommend an aggressive pumping program of 1 to 3 days, 8 to 10 hours per day, in order to maximize the effect of treatment and limit patient inconvenience. Maximal results of pumping can usually be achieved during this time period, and the therapist avoids the problem of long-term patient compliance. After pumping, the individual is fitted with a custom compression garment to maintain the reduction. This is followed by a serial sleeving program involving the application of progressively smaller sleeves every 4 to 6 weeks. When this technique is used, the garment acts as a compression dressing rather than a device to merely maintain the achieved reduction.

If patient compliance for a pumping program is not possible, serial sleeving is a viable option—it simply requires more time. I suggest ordering a sleeve that is 2 to 3 mm smaller than the actual circumferential measurements to ensure that the sleeve acts dynamically to reduce the patient's edema. In my experience, about 10 to 15 percent of patients with edema can be completely weaned from their garment and instructed in a self-monitoring program, 40 percent require regular use of a sleeve on some basis to maintain good reduction of pain and edema, 30 percent require the use of the sleeve at all times to control their edema, and the remainder have a poor response to treatment. It is important to be aware that a patient who once develops edema following resolution is more likely to have another exacerbation than one with no prior history of edema.

There are other compression techniques that can be utilized for specific problems, particularly those involving the hands. Examples include use of gloves, other compression wrapping, electrical stimulation, water submersion, icing, and Plastazote pads. These items are selected for particular problems and require therapists to be well versed in this area. It is not within the scope of this chapter to discuss these in detail.

Functional Outcome/Quality of Life

In terms of physical therapy management, individuals with breast cancers can benefit from treatment intervention. Therapists can help to maintain mobility, to decrease pain, and to achieve a more acceptable cosmetic effect; they can also provide adaptive equipment as necessary and educate patients to monitor and assess their own status. The nature of the physical therapist's work requires constant invasion of patients' personal space, touching them where they may be reluctant to touch themselves. This precious aspect of the care given by the therapist provides a vehicle for patients to express their concerns, to ask questions, to verbalize their fears, and to discuss adjustments to their jobs, families and significant others. It is a privileged communication to which the therapist must respond in a positive but realistic manner, cautioning patients to expect the worst—because they do have a life-threatening disease—and to hope for the best—because people are survivors by nature.

REFERENCES

1. Haagensen CD: Diseases of the Breast. 3rd Ed. WB Saunders, Philadelphia, 1986, p. 976
2. Case C (ed): The Breast Cancer Digest. 2nd Ed. U.S. Department of Health and Human Services, National Institutes of Health 1984, p. 1
3. Lichter AS, Lippman ME: Special situations in the treatment of breast cancer. p. 407. In Lippman, ME, Lichter AS, Danforth DN (eds): Diagnosis and Management of Breast Cancer. WB Sauders Philadelphia, 1988
4. Silverberg E, Lubera JA: Cancer statistics. CA 39(1):9, 1989
5. Wilson JD, Griffin J: Disorders of sexual differentiation. p. 724. In Petersdorf RG, Adams RD, Braunwald E, et al. (eds): Harrison's Principles of Internal Medicine. 10th Ed. McGraw-Hill, New York, 1983

6. Townsend CM: Management of breast cancer surgery and adjuvant therapy. Clin Symp 39(4):3, 1987

7. Henderson IC: Breast Cancer Management Progress and Prospects. Lederle Laboratories, Wayne NJ, 1984

8. Fisher B, Slack N, Katrych D, et al: Ten year follow-up results of patients with carcinoma of the breast in a cooperative clinical trial evaluating surgical adjuvant chemotherapy. Surg Gynecol Obstet 140:528, 1975

9. Townsend CM: Breast lumps. Clin Symp 32(2):16, 1980

10. Furmanski P, Saunders DE, Brooks SL, et al: Prognostic value of estrogen receptor determinations in patients with primary breast cancer, an update. Cancer 46: 2794, 1980

11. Haagensen CD: Diseases of the Breast. 3rd Ed. WB Saunders, Philadelphia, 1986, p. 866

12. Haagensen CD: Diseases of the Breast. 3rd Ed. WB Saunders, Philadelphia, 1986, p. 940

13. Danforth DN, Lippman ME: Surgical treatment of breast cancer. p. 95. In Lippman ME, Lichter AS, Danforth DN (eds): Diagnosis and Management of Breast Cancer. WB Saunders, Philadelphia, 1988

14. Del Regato JA, Spjut HJ: Ackerman and del Regato's Cancer Diagnosis, Treatment, and Prognosis. 5th Ed. CV Mosby, St. Louis, 1977, p. 850

15. Lichter AS, Findlay PA: Radiation therapy as an adjuvant to surgery in the treatment of operable breast cancer. p. 228. In Lippman ME, Lichter AS, Danforth ND (eds): Diagnosis and Management of Breast Cancer. WB Saunders, Philadelphia, 1988

16. Woll JE: Breast Cancer. p. 179. In Rosenthal S, Carignan JR, Smith BD (eds): Medical Care of the Cancer Patient. WB Saunders, Philadelphia, 1987

17. Britton RC, Nelson PA: Causes and treatment of postmastectomy lymphedema of the arm. JAMA 180:95, 1962

18. Wittlinger G, Wittlinger H: Introduction to Dr. Vodder's Manual Lymph Drainage. Vol. 1. Haug Publishers, Heidelberg, 1982, p. 23

5 | Rehabilitation of the Leukemia/Lymphoma Patient

Lauren Holtzman
Kathleen Chesney

LEUKEMIA

The term *leukemia* represents a group of diseases characterized by "unregulated proliferation and incomplete maturation of the precursors to white cells and lymphocytes."[1] This results in a high white count, with a large number of immature cells, or blasts, in the peripheral blood and bone marrow. There will also be a lowered red cell and platelet count due to the lack of space in the bone marrow and the disruption of the blood-forming system. The exact presentation of blood counts and types of cells will depend on the type of leukemia with which the patient has been diagnosed. There are four major types; acute myelogenous leukemia, acute lymphoblastic leukemia, chronic myelogenous leukemia and chronic lymphocytic leukemia.[1]

HEMATOPOIESIS

In order to understand the mechanism of leukemia, one must understand hematopoiesis, the mechanism by which the bone marrow forms red cells, white cells, platelets, and lymphocytes. Hematopoiesis can be divided into five distinct levels. The first level is the stem cell, the most primitive of cells. This cell is called *pluripotent* as it is the progenitor of all lymphopoiesis and hematopoiesis.

85

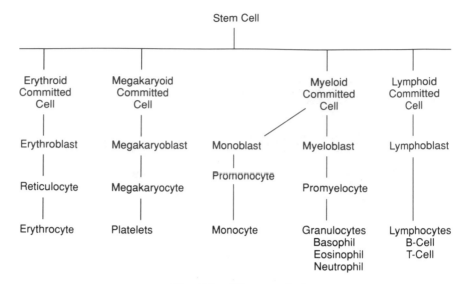

Fig. 5-1. Hematopoiesis.

At the second level the stem cell divides into two separate stem cell pools, hematopoietic cells, which are the precursors of the six types of blood cells, and lymphopoietic stem cells, which are the precursors of lymphoid cells. The third level is where differentiation takes place with formation of committed progenitor cells. These are termed *unipotential* and become one of the six types of blood cells or one of two lymphocytes. The precursors of blood cells are formed at the fourth level; these are known as the *committed progenitors*. At level five the precursor cells undergo maturation to form mature functional blood cells.[1] This process is depicted in Fig. 5-1.

In leukemic hematopoiesis there is a proliferation of cells derived from a leukemic pluripotent or hematopoietic stem cell. These cells either do not mature or mature defectively. The percentage of cells dividing and the total time it takes to complete the cell cycle are usually the same as or can even be less than that of normal hematopoietic cells. The total number of primitive cells is increased because they do not mature. As the defect is in the stem cell, red cells and platelets may also be affected.[1]

ETIOLOGY

In many cases the exact cause of leukemia cannot be identified; however, there are many possible influencing factors.

1. *Environmental factors:* Exposure to high-dose radiation has been associated with an increased incidence of leukemia, as seen after the dropping of the nuclear bomb on Hiroshima and the nuclear accident at Chernobyl, as well as after radiation treatment for other malignancies such as Hodgkin's disease.[1,2]

2. *Genetic factors:* Certain of these are associated with high risk for the development of leukemia, as in Down syndrome, Bloom syndrome, Fanconi's anemia, Kleinfelter syndrome.[1,3]

3. *Viral factors:* These have been identified in animal leukemias, and certain viruses (HTLVI and HTLVII) have been isolated as possible causes of human leukemia.[1,3]

4. *Immunologic factors:* Some research suggests that a defect in the immune system may increase the possibility of a neoplasm.[1]

It is important to remember that in most cases of leukemia a causative factor cannot be identified.

DIAGNOSTIC PROCEDURES

Leukemia is diagnosed initially by peripheral blood cell counts. Peripheral blood smears will identify anemia, thrombocytopenia, and an abnormal white blood cell count. White blood count may be high or low but will show an abnormal number of immature cells.

To definitively diagnose leukemia a bone marrow biopsy and aspiration are carried out. A sample of bone marrow is taken from the posteior iliac crest and evaluated under a microscope. In this way the type of leukemia can be identified by the type of immature cells present in the bone marrow.[1]

TYPES OF LEUKEMIA

Acute Myelogenous Leukemia

Acute myelogenous leukemia (AML) may also be termed acute nonlymphoblastic leukemia (ANLL).[4] In AML there is an accumulation of myeloblasts and other immature myeloid cells. The bone marrow is invaded by these malignant cells, which disrupts normal hematopoiesis.[5] In children less than 15 years of age 17 percent of all leukemia cases are AML. In children AML has an extremely poor prognosis even with treatment.[4] In adults there are 3 cases per 100,000 population and approximately 7,000 cases per year in the United States. Without treatment the median survival is less than 2 months. Death results from hemorrhage or infection.[5]

Clinical Signs and Physical Findings

Symptoms of anemia include feelings of fatigue, dyspnea on exertion, palpitations, and pallor.[4,5] Neutropenia, or low mature white cell count, results in local infection, fever, and chills. Low platelet count, known as *thrombocytopenia,* presents as bleeding of the gums, gastrointestinal tract, or urinary tract, or simply as superficial cutaneous bleeding. In general the patient may feel fatigue and general malaise and, rarely, joint pain.[5]

On physical examination one may note pallor, small areas of bleeding, enlarged liver and spleen, and, rarely, enlarged lymph nodes. Occasionally a localized tumor may arise from organ infiltration by leukemic cells.[5]

Classification

While staging procedures are not appropriate in the diagnosis of AML, there are seven classifications that influence the disease prognosis. Figure 5-1 may be used to identify the predominant cell lines. M1, *acute differentiated myelocytic leukemia*, is identified by the predominance of myeloblasts. In M2, *acute undifferentiated myelocytic* leukemia, the cells are mainly myeloblasts and promyelocytes that mature abnormally. M3, *acute promyelocytic leukemia*, presents mainly with promyelocytes. In M4, *acute myelomonocytic leukemia*, the predominant cells are promyelocytes, myelocytes, promonocytes, and monocytes, and some cell maturation is evident in the peripheral blood. M5 is divided into A and B subclasses: M5A, *acute monoblastic leukemia*, presents with undifferentiated or primitive monoblasts; M5B, *acute differentiated monocytic leukemia*, displays more mature cells, with promonocytes and monocytes also present. M6, *acute erythroleukemia*, affects the red cell line, with erythroblasts predominant. In M7, which affects the platelet precursors and is termed *megakaryocytic leukemia*, the cells resemble those of M1, but there is fibrosis of bone marrow.[4,5] The prognosis worsens and the chance for remission decreases as the classification number increases.

Acute Lymphoblastic Leukemia

Acute lymphoblastic leukemia (ALL) is characterized by the proliferation of immature lymphocytes and their precursors.[6] The disease may be present in the central nervous system (CNS). ALL is most common in children, accounting for 83 percent of all childhood leukemias.[4] In adults the incidence is lower, but ALL still represents a large number of leukemia cases.[3,4] There are 6 new cases per 100,000 population.[1]

Clinical Signs and Physical Findings

Patients will experience malaise, lethargy, fatigue, loss of appetite, abdominal discomfort, and headache. They may have fever; bleeding from gums, skin, or nose; and liver, spleen, or testicular enlargement. Bone and joint pain are common symptoms.

On examination patients will present with pallor, small areas of bleeding on the skin, and liver and spleen enlargement. Organ infiltration may occur from leukemic cells; cells may invade the cerebrospinal fluid, leading to leukemic meningitis or CNS disease, which present as headache, mental status change, diplopia, cranial nerve palsy, and papilledema.[1,5]

Classification

ALL can be divided into three subtypes, L1, L2, and L3. In L1 cells are small, with a small amount of cytoplasm and indistinct nuclei; 85 percent of ALL in children is of this subtype. L2 presents with large cells, more cytoplasm, and prominent nuclei and is mostly seen in adults. L3, in which the cells resemble those of Burkitt's lymphoma, represents less than 1 percent of all cases, occasionally presents in adults, and has most recently been seen in patients with the acquired immunodeficiency syndrome (AIDS).[1,2,6,7]

In a second method of classification, based on the immunologic type of lymphoblast,[1] the subtype is assigned on the basis of T-cell or B-cell markers; if neither marker is present, the ALL is considered to be of the null-cell type. Certain null-cell types have been subtyped common ALL because they react to an antibody made from an antigen commonly found in ALL cells.[1,2,6,7]

Chronic Myelogenous Leukemia

Chronic myelogenous leukemia (CML) presents with a proliferation of myeloid cells and their precursors. This is usually accompanied by a Philadelphia chromosome, which is a translocation of the long arms of chromosome 22 to another chromosome. Initially the predominant cells in the marrow are mature or partially mature, but this changes in time.[1,8] During the first year the disease remains in this form, and it may stay this way for years. Without treatment median survival is 3 to 5 years; less than 30 percent of patients survive 5 years.[8] CML is not common before the age of 20; but its incidence increases with age. Males show a greater predisposition to this type of leukemia than females.[1]

Clinical Signs and Physical Findings

Initial symptoms include malaise, fatigue, sweating, heat intolerance, susceptibility to bruising, abdominal discomfort, and an enlarged spleen. On examination, bruising, cutaneous bleeding, gum bleeding, spleen enlargement, and occasionally a tumor of myeloblasts may be found.[1]

Classification

CML presents in three separate phases. The first, or chronic phase, during which some myeloid cells mature normally, is unstable, and transformation to one of the other phases eventually occurs. In the second, acute phase, or blast crisis, the disease becomes more aggressive and begins to resemble an acute leukemia[8]; blast transformation can occur along myeloid or lymphoid lines.[1] In the third, or accelerated phase, symptoms progress, resulting in an increased resistance to treatment.[8]

Chronic Lymphocytic Leukemia

Chronic lymphocytic leukemia (CLL) is characterized by proliferation of "mature-appearing" lymphocytes,[9] which are long-lived and therefore accumulate in the bone marrow, blood, lymph nodes, liver, and spleen.[1] This disease usually occurs in patients over 50 years of age and is the most common form of leukemia in adults.[9]

The clinical course of this disease can be quite variable. Certain patients will not require therapy, as the disease may not be life-threatening. Conversely, some patients may have a rapid, progressive course and a projected survival of less than 2 years.[9]

Clinical Signs and Physical Findings

Patients will present with malaise, fatigue, weight loss, excessive sweating, and abdominal discomfort from enlarged organs. Initially patients can present with skin infection or pneumonia and lymph adenopathy.[1] On physical examination enlarged lymph nodes and possibly an enlarged spleen and liver will be found, as well as skin infiltrates. Anemia of varying degrees and a low platelet count may also occur.[1]

Classification

CLL can initially be stable for several months and then be transformed into a more aggressive form of the disease.[9] Once transformed, it can be classified into one of three types. B-cell CLL is similar to poorly differentiated lymphoma and has a more aggressive course. T-cell CLL is found in less than 5 percent of cases of well differentiated lymphocytic lymphoma; these lymphocytes are of T-cell phenotype. Prolymphocytic leukemia is a variant of CLL with a poorer prognosis and can eventually progress to an acute, or blast crisis.[1,9]

Other Types of Leukemia

There are other types of leukemia that are lymphocytic in nature, including hairy cell, plasma cell, Sézary cell, and lymphoma cell leukemia. These are less common than the four major types of leukemia previously described.[1]

ANTINEOPLASTIC TREATMENT

The main form of treatment for leukemia is chemotherapy. The purpose of the treatment is to obtain a complete remission (CR), defined as less than 5 percent blasts or immature cells in the bone marrow, in hope of an eventual cure. Various factors affect the achievement and maintenance of a CR: (1) age—usually younger patients fare better; (2) sex—females have a better prognosis; (3) performance status—the higher, the better; (4) normal organ function; (5) low blast count on diagnosis; (6) high platelet count; (7) absence of leukemia in other areas of the body; (8) high sensitivity to drugs in vitro; (9) rapid decrease in blast cells and rapid time to CR; (10) few chemotherapy cycles to CR.[5]

Treatment of AML

Treatment of AML consists of an induction phase, in which the goal is to induce a CR, and an augmentation stage designed to prolong the remission, usually started approximately 6 weeks after recovery from induction.[5,10] Maintenance chemotherapy (i.e., use of lower doses of the same drugs used for induction therapy for 2 to 3 years to maintain remission) and intensification, or postremission treatment, 6 months after induction treatment are not generally used in the treatment of adults with AML. However, it may be of benefit in the treatment of children.[5]

The most effective chemotherapy agents are cytosine arabinoside (ara-C), daunorubicin, and m-amsacrine (amsa).[10] When these are used as single agents, a 25 to 50 percent remission rate can be achieved, and when they are used in combination, a 65 to 85 percent remission rate is possible.[5] The incidence of central nervous system (CNS) involvement is between 5 and 20 percent, and the treatment of choice is usually ara-C or methotrexate although there is no evidence that this increases long-term survival.[5] In general, the prognosis is better for adults than children.[4]

Treatment of ALL

The optimum therapy for childhood ALL is vincristine and prednisone, which have resulted in CR rates of 83 to 95 percent. If L-asparaginase is added to the combination, 90 to 95 percent CR rates are achieved. Historically, 50 to 70 percent of children with ALL will develop CNS leukemia if untreated. Many patients will receive chemotherapy or radiation to prevent CNS dysfunction. Children will receive maintenance therapy for 3 years to maintain remission.[4]

The optimum treatment for ALL in adults consists of prednisone and vincristine added to ara-C and daunorubinicin, resulting in a 75 to 80 percent remission rate. Remissions in adults are short, typically lasting 11 to 19 months. The incidence of CNS disease is less than 10 percent, and the effect of preventive treatment has been controversial.[6]

Treatment of CML

Initial treatment of CML in the chronic phase includes the use of busulfan or hydroxyurea. These drugs suppress the progress of the disease but do not cure it. Once the disease has entered the acute or accelerated phase, it is treated with the same agents used for ALL, sometimes with the addition of interferon.

The prognosis for patients who enter the acute or accelerated phase is poor, resulting in short remissions and low chance of long-term survival. Bone marrow transplantation offers a 63 percent disease-free survival when it is done in the chronic phase, 36 percent in the accelerated phase, and 12 percent in the acute phase.[7] Bone marrow transplantation, considered the only cure for CML,[11] will be discussed in detail later in this chapter.

Side Effects of Treatment

The side effects of chemotherapy or radiation treatment influence clinical course and physical therapy intervention. The major side effect of chemotherapy is myelosuppression, or lowered blood counts, which is severe in the treatment of leukemia, as the bone marrow is the site of the disease. Other side effects are nausea and vomiting and hair loss. In addition specific toxicities of certain agents affect the clinical course. Ara-C increases the risk of pulmonary capillary leak syndrome, which can lead to adult respiratory distress syndrome (ARDS). In order to prevent this, patients are placed on fluid restriction, which results in dehydration and orthostatic hypotension. Patients are placed on bed rest for of 1 to 2 weeks to prevent injury from falling or fainting.[10] Amsa has cardiotoxic effects, which may lead to arrhythmias.[10] Vincristine has been found to cause peripheral neuropathies, specifically in the peroneal and radial nerves, causing sensory and motor deficits. Prednisone is a steroid, which with prolonged use can lead to proximal muscle weakness and aseptic necrosis of hips or shoulders, as well as to joint pain upon withdrawal of the drug.[12] Toxic effects of CNS therapy include neuropsychologic effects and encephalopathy.[4] All these effects will affect the role of the physical therapist in treating the leukemia patient.

PHYSICAL THERAPY INTERVENTION

Specific physical therapy intervention is dependent on the patient's diagnosis, therapy received, age, and treatment course. The first course of action is preventive. The average length of stay in the hospital is 4 to 5 weeks,[10,12] and as a result of this prolonged hospitalization, patients with AML and ALL are at risk for loss of strength and endurance and may develop osteoporosis due to the secondary effects of bed rest. In addition, nausea and vomiting from chemotherapy will restrict activity for a time. It is important, therefore, to educate patients and to provide them with an exercise program that includes active exercise and walking. When designing an exercise program, it is important to remember the myelosuppressive action of the chemotherapeutic agents. Low white cell counts place patients at risk for infection and are accompanied by high fevers, making exercise difficult. Low platelet counts place patients at risk for bleeding, and therefore resistive exercise is rarely used. A low hematocrit can lead to intolerance of activity. Vital signs, including pulse and respiratory rate, must be closely monitored during exercise and activity.

The side effects of other drugs may further complicate the clinical course, and patients may require more intensive intervention. The major side effect of ara-C, as previously stated, is the increased risk for ARDS. These patients are fluid-restricted, which leads to severe orthostatic hypotension, a condition that becomes more serious for the elderly patient. Bed rest for up to 2 weeks is mandatory for these patients to prevent falls and injury. During this time patients can only tolerate very gentle bedside exercise owing to low blood volume. The result is a significant loss of strength and endurance, which leads to difficulty in ambulation and activities of daily living. A small percentage of patients will experience continued orthostasis and balance impairment after the fluid has been replaced. These patients require a program geared toward rehabilitation, which may include a therapeutic exercise program, endurance training, progressive elevation activities, and gait training.

Patients who receive vincristine are at risk for developing peroneal palsy and radial wrist drop. These neuropathies will resolve on their own after 1 to 2 years, but certain measures need to be taken to preserve function and prevent contractures. Patients should be splinted, instructed in appropriate stretching exercises, and provided with a molded ankle and foot orthosis to improve gait and safety.

There is a group of patients who may not achieve a remission after many courses of chemotherapy. These patients may be very debilitated by the side effects of treatment and by multiple infections and complications. Their life expectancy may be only weeks to a few months. The focus of treatment in these patients is to help them to maximize function and to teach the family to help care for them so that they may maintain quality of life and be able to achieve any goals they wish.

BONE MARROW TRANSPLANTATION

Bone marrow transplantation (BMT) is becoming the preferred form of treatment for many forms of cancer, especially the more resistant forms of leukemia and lymphoma in patients under 50 years of age. Currently there are approximately 35 active BMT units in the United States.[13]

There are three basic types of BMT:

1. Allogeneic: the bone marrow is donated by a human leukocyte antigen (HLA)-matched donor, usually a sibling.
2. Syngeneic: the bone marrow is donated by an identical twin.
3. Autologous: when the patient's own bone marrow is reinfused after being harvested and treated.[13]

Each type of BMT has its complications and risks.

Treatment Procedures

The preparative treatment is similar regardless of the disease being treated or the kind of BMT being done. Treatment consists of 4 days of high-dose chemotherapy, usually with Cytoxan, and 4 days of total body irradiation. In some cases a second course of high-dose chemotherapy (usually with busulfan) will be used instead of total body irradiation.[13,14] In an autologous BMT the patient's bone marrow will be removed from the posterior iliac crest and then treated with the chemotherapeutic agent 4-hydroperoxycyclophosphamide (4-HC)[15] prior to the preparative regimen. The preparative regimen kills the tumor cells and destroys the bone marrow. The marrow is then reinfused, usually via an atrial line.[13] The transplantation is followed by a 3- to 4-week period of aplasia or immunosuppression, in which the white blood cell count is below 1,000/mm.[3] During this time patients are confined to the nursing floor.[16] The minimum hospital stay for these patients is approximately 6 weeks.[16]

Complications

There are many complications that can interfere with a patient's course. Infection can occur as a result of prolonged immunosuppression and is a typical problem in all types of BMT. Patients are at risk for lung infection caused by bacterial, viral, or fungal organisms or secondary to blood infections or urinary or gastrointestinal tract infections.[15,17] Despite vigorous treatment, infection can lead to death in the immunosuppressed patient. Interstitial pneumonitis is the cause of 40 percent of transplant-related deaths. Patients develop interstitial infiltrates, edema, fibrosis, cellular infiltrates, and alveolar exudates. In 60 percent of the cases the cause of death is unknown but may be an undiagnosed infection. Other cases are attributed to lung infection, especially by cytomegalovirus.[17]

Hepatic veno-occlusive disease is the obliteration of the small intrahepatic central venules. There is no known treatment for this disease, which can progress to renal failure.[13] *Mucositis* is oral ulceration and hemorrhage caused by chemotherapy and immunosuppression. It is an extremely painful condition, often requiring morphine for symptomatic relief.[13]

Graft-versus-host disease (GVHD) is a side effect usually seen with an allogeneic BMT and rarely seen in autologous or syngeneic transplants. GVHD is the largest cause of death in patients and has a 33 percent fatality rate.[18] Its overall incidence in BMT cases is 40 to 60 percent. Acute GVHD occurs when the graft or donor's bone marrow reacts against the patient's body systems. Target organs are the skin, liver, and gastrointestinal tract. Patients are treated prophylactically with cyclosporin A and steroids if the disease becomes active.[13] Acute GVHD progresses to the chronic form in at least 50 percent of patients. Symptoms include fibrosis of skin, fascia, liver, and bowel; if the disease is left untreated it may lead to contractures. Treatment includes steroids and immunosuppressive therapy.[18]

Relapse or reoccurrence of disease is the largest cause of death in syngeneic and autologous BMTs.

Results

The success of a BMT depends on the disease being treated and at what point in the progression of the disease the patient receives the transplant.

Patients with leukemia have a better prognosis if the transplant is received in the first or second remission.[13,15,19–21] Those with CML should receive it in the chronic rather than the acute or accelerated phase.[11] In the first remission with AML there is a 40 to 70 percent and in the second remission a 20 to 25 percent long-term survival rate. Among patients with ALL there is a 30 to 50 percent long-term survival rate in first remission and a 25 to 35 percent rate in second or third remission. Patients with CML receiving transplants in the chronic phase have a 50 to 60 percent chance of long-term survival, compared with only a 15 to 30 percent chance in accelerated or acute phase.[13] Patients diagnosed with CLL are typically not candidates for BMT because of older age.[8]

There is some controversy regarding treatment of Hodgkin's disease and non-Hodgkin's lymphoma with BMT. The Johns Hopkins group reports a 50 percent disease-free survival rate and a 40 percent relapse rate. Patients who had "bulky" tumors, defined as those larger than 5 cm, had a lower chance of survival.[15] However, other researchers feel that in view of the success of chemotherapy and radiation in the treatment of lymphomas and the mortality rate in BMT, its use in first remission is not warranted and that it should be considered only after patients have failed first-line chemotherapy.[22]

Physical Therapy Intervention

All patients who are to undergo BMT should be placed on a comprehensive exercise program to prevent loss of strength and endurance as well as to maintain mobility and thus prevent lung infection by aiding in the clearing of secretions.[6]

Certain considerations must be taken into account when designing an exercise program. First, treatment of GVHD requires high-dose steroids, which place patients at risk of aseptic necrosis, osteoporosis, and steroid myopathies. Upper extremity weight bearing, back extension, and ambulation, as well as proximal muscle strengthening, are essential to every exercise program. Second, the myelosuppressive action of chemotherapy necessitates monitoring blood counts closely. This includes avoiding resistive exercise when platelet counts are lower than $50,000/mm^3$, and avoiding all activity when counts are lower than $20,000/mm^3$, a time when risk of intracranial hemorrhage is high. A low hematocrit requires monitoring of vital signs (pulse rate and respiration) and may require modification of the exercise program if exercise tolerance decreases.

In addition to these considerations, complications may further debilitate the patient, resulting in the need for intubation, dialysis, or simply prolonged bed rest. Intracranial bleeding may result in neurologic deficits, causing weakness and loss of motor control and equilibrium. These deficits may be a result of prolonged bed rest or focal infarct. The physical therapy program must then focus on range of motion, balance, strengthening, endurance, and progressive ambulation in order to restore function.

Early physical therapy intervention allows the therapist to follow patients closely to monitor changes in physical and medical status and therefore provide services as soon as necessary.

LYMPHOMA

In 1832 Thomas Hodgkin described seven cases of enlarged lymph nodes not believed to be caused by inflammation, thereby marking the first recognition of the malignant lymphomas as a clinical entity. Hodgkin's disease, *lymphosarcoma*, and leukemia were distinguished as separate diagnoses toward the end of the nineteenth century. Since then cancers of the lymphoreticular system, a very heterogeneous group, have seen ongoing subclassification.[23] Lymphomas are malignant tumors that arise from the cellular elements of the lymph nodes, bone marrow, and occasionally other organs having a reticuloendothelial content. These cells destroy the normal architecture of the lymph nodes. Generally originating at a single site, they can spread to other lymph nodes and subsequently become disseminated to the spleen, liver, bone marrow, lungs, and other sites.[24] Two major categories of lymphoma are recognized, Hodgkin's disease and the non-Hodgkin's lymphomas. Although the signs and symptoms of the lymphomas may overlap, the treatment and prognosis for each kind are different. Thus, it is absolutely essential to establish an accurate diagnosis so that the optimal treatment can be delivered. The lymphomas are differentiated according to the predominant types of cells found in the lymph nodes as well as by their growth pattern (nodular or diffuse).[25] After tissue diagnosis has been established by surgical removal and microscopic study of one or more lymph nodes, staging procedures are conducted to determine the extent of disease. From these results treatment and prognosis can then be established.

The progress made in treatment of lymphomas is notable, for it is in the treatment of these malignancies that it was first shown that chemotherapy could cure a significant number of the adult population affected by cancer of a major organ system. Because of advances in treatment since the middle to late 1960s, lymphomas, once considered universally fatal, are often cured or substantially palliated. Over 70 percent of HD patients are curable, as are 50 to 60 percent of NHL patients overall.[26,27]

HODGKIN'S DISEASE

Incidence and Etiology

Hodgkin's disease (HD) accounts for about 40 percent of the malignant lymphomas, making it the most common form of this type of cancer. In 1986 there were 8,000 new cases of HD. It affects predominantly young and middle-aged adults, with about 50 percent of cases occurring between ages 20 and 40 years. Onset after age 60 is seen in fewer than 10 percent of cases, and fewer than 10 percent of cases occur before age 10. There is a male/female predominance of 4 : 2.6, males having a poorer prognosis.[23,26]

The cause of HD is unknown. Reports of clusters of cases as well as of an increased incidence among family members has established the possibility of an infectious factor. The association of HD with certain HLA antigens points to genetic factors as well. Infectivity and genetic factors may be interrelated, as viral transmission and the susceptibility of certain individuals to oncogenic agents may be influenced by genetic factors.[28] Of note is the fact that HD patients, both those untreated and those examined after complete remission of disease and cessation of treatment, show abnormalities in their cellular immunity, as demonstrated by delayed hypersensitivity skin testing and lymphocyte transformation in vitro. These aberrations range from minor to complete anergy and may influence the HD patient's susceptibility to infectious complications such as herpes zoster and *Pneumocystis carinii* infection and perhaps their susceptibility to HD itself.[23,29]

Classification

The presence of the Reed-Sternberg cell, a malignant type of histiocyte (tissue macrophage), is essential for the diagnosis of HD. This is a large bi- or multinucleated cell containing large nucleoli and is considered to be derived

Table 5-1. Histopathologic Classification of Hodgkin's Disease—1966 Ryc Conference[23,29]

Lymphocytic predominance
  About 5 percent of the total
  Abundant normal lymphocytes and small
    numbers of Reed-Sternberg cells
  Occurs in both nodular and diffuse forms
  Is the least aggressive histologic form of the
    disease

Nodular sclerosis
  About 50 percent of most series
  Nodules of abnormal lymphoid tissue
  Nodules are surrounded by annular bands of
    collagen extending from a dense capsule
  RS cells are very large, lacunar variant

Mixed cellularity
  37 percent of the total
  Pleocellular infiltrate with a background of
    plasma cells, neutrophils, eosinophils,
    lymphocytes, and histiocytes
  Moderate numbers of Reed-Steinberg cells
  Fibrosis, if present, is disorderly and
    without collagen formation

Lymphocytic depletion
  Lymphocytes rare or absent
  Many Reed-Sternberg cells
  Is the most malignant histologic form of the
    disease

from the interdigitating reticular cell of lymph nodes.[30] HD affects the lymph nodes first, replacing them with tumors that consist of reticular cells together with lymphocytes, granulocytes, plasma cells, and fibroblasts.[24,30] It can spread later to involve almost any organ.[1] Histologically HD can be divided into four subtypes according to the Rye classification system (Table 5-1).

Staging

The 1971 Ann Arbor system is used for clinical and pathologic staging of HD (Table 5-2). Pathologic staging is based on surgical sampling of tissues during laparotomy.

Clinical Features

Presentation is typically characterized by painless lymph node involvement, with or without constitutional (B) symptoms. Lymphadenopathy occurs supradiaphragmatically 90 percent of the time, with cervical nodes affected in 60 to 80 percent of cases. Axillary or mediastinal presentations are much less common; mediastinal lymphadenopathy can cause cough, dyspnea, or superior vena cava obstruction. In only about 10 percent of cases does presentation involve inguinal or abdominal masses. If the disease becomes generalized, then involvement of the retroperitoneal nodes, spleen, liver, and/or bone marrow will occur in most cases.[23,29]

Table 5-2. Hodgkin's Disease: Ann Arbor Clinical Staging Classification[a]

Stage	Definition
Stage I	Involvement of a single lymph node region (I) or of a single extralymphatic organ or site (I_E)
Stage II	Involvement of two or more lymph node regions on same side of diaphragm (II) *or* Localized involvement of an extralymphatic organ or site and of one or more lymph node regions on same side of diaphragm (II_E)
Stage III	Involvement of lymph node regions on both sides of the diaphragm (III), which may also be accompanied by involvement of the spleen (III_S) or by localized involvement of an extralymphatic organ or site (III_E) or by both (III_{SE})
Stage IV	Diffuse or disseminated involvement of one or more extralymphatic organs or tissues, with or without associated lymph node involvement
	Biopsy-documented involvement of stage IV sites is also denoted by letter suffixes: marrow = M+, lung = L+, liver (hepatic) = H+, pleura = P+, bone (osseous) = O+, skin and subcutaneous tissue (dermal) = D+.
	The presence or absence of fever, night sweats, and/or unexplained weight loss of 10 percent or more of body weight in the 6 months preceding admission is denoted by the suffix letters B and A, respectively.

[a] Adopted at the Workshop on the Staging of Hodgkin's Disease held at Ann Arbor, Michigan in April 1971.[31]

(From Kaplan,[31] with permission.)

HD appears to be of unifocal origin and spreads via lymph channels in a sequential manner to contiguous nodal areas. Further dissemination once the spleen becomes involved probably occurs via the bloodstream.[23,29,31] The predictable contiguous spread pattern is a distinctive characteristic of HD, whereas in NHL nodes and bone marrow are more often involved in less predictable patterns. In HD the radiation oncologist is therefore able to predict the lymph nodes that are highly likely to have microscopic disease and to include them in radiation treatment.

Antineoplastic Treatment

Surgery

Staging laparotomy, which provides information to determine the pathologic stage, is the primary role of surgery in HD patients. It is usually indicated in all but stage IV patients and provides for more accurate evaluation than does clinical staging as the pathologic stage has been found to differ from the clinical stage in 30 percent of patients.[23,29] The exploratory laparotomy includes systemic sampling of all lymph node groups, bone marrow biopsy, liver biopsies, and splenectomy; it is used to rule out visceral involvement before extensive lymph node irradiation is begun (because if the disease is disseminated chemotherapy alone would be the treatment of choice). In females the ovaries are transposed out of the radiation field at the time of this surgery.[23,29]

Radiation Therapy

Intensive megavoltage radiation therapy is the treatment of choice for all patients with localized stages of HD (stages I, II, and some IIIA). When nodes are very large or B symptoms are present, chemotherapy may be used along with radiation therapy. Radiation therapy to eradicate HD demands a dosage of about 3,500 to 4,500 rads, which is delivered over 4 to 8 weeks at about 150 to 200 rads per fraction of treatment. It is essential that extended-field irradiation be used so as to include the contiguous clinically uninvolved nodal sites and thus ensure a high probability of complete cure. Total nodal irradiation to encompass the entire axial lymph node system may be carried out. Protection of the lungs, spinal cord, larynx, heart, kidneys, gonads, and iliac crest marrow is provided by field shaping and shielding.[23,29,31]

Chemotherapy

Chemotherapy is always the primary mode of treatment for patients with stage IV disease. The presence of B symptoms in stage II and III patients indicates a worse prognosis than does their absence. In order to maximize the chance for CR in these patients (the only reasonable chance of cure will be in those who achieve a CR), most stage IIB patients are treated with either extended field or total nodal irradiation along with chemotherapy; stage IIIB patients receive total nodal irradiation and chemotherapy.[23,27,29]

The use of combination chemotherapy for treatment of advanced HD began in 1964 when DeVita et al. developed the four-drug combination nitrogen mustard-Oncovin-procarbazine-prednisone (MOPP) (see Table 5-3). This regimen was chosen on the basis of the antitumor activity of each agent when used alone and to minimize overlapping toxicity among the drugs to any single organ.

Table 5-3. Selected Combination Chemotherapy Regimens in Advanced Hodgkin's Disease and Non-Hodgkin's Lymphoma

Acronym	Drugs
MOPP	Nitrogen *M*ustard *O*ncovin (vincristine) *P*rocarbazine *P*rednisone
ABVD	*A*driamycin (doxorubicin) *B*leomycin *V*elban *D*acarbazine
C-MOPP	*C*ytoxan (cyclophosphamide) Followed by MOPP
CHOP	*C*ytoxan *H*ydroxydaunorubicin *O*ncovin *P*rednisone
M-BACOD	*M*ethotrexate *B*leomycin *A*driamycin *C*ytoxan *O*ncovin *D*examethasone
MACOP-B	*M*ethotrexate *A*driamycin *C*ytoxan *O*ncovin *P*rednisone *B*leomycin
ProMACE-MOPP	*P*rednisone *V*P-16 *M*ethotrexate *A*driamycin *C*ytoxan Followed by MOPP

(From Skarin et al,[30] with permission.)

Over a 2-week period these four drugs are given to their full dose; this is followed by a 2-week recovery period to permit resolution of myelosuppression. A minimum of six cycles is given in this manner until CR is attained or tumor growth occurs in spite of treatment.[26]

Other drugs were found with antitumor activity against this cancer. Bonadonna et al. developed a new drug combination, Adriamycin-bleomycin-Velban-dacarbazine (ABVD) (Table 5-3), as a salvage treatment for patients refractory to MOPP. These drugs were selected partly because of their different mechanisms of action compared with MOPP. This new combination demonstrated effectiveness equal to MOPP; however, ABVD is generally not used for the initial induction because of the potential cardiopulmonary toxicity of doxorubicin (Adriamycin) and bleomycin.[23,27] A regimen alternating one course of MOPP with one course of ABVD has been reported to have a slightly higher CR rate than MOPP alone.[23,26,27] This regimen has been primarily used for patients with advanced disease stage III or IV.[27]

Maintenance therapy provides no benefit to HD patients once an intensive CR-inducing regimen has been completed.[23] Single-agent chemotherapy can be used to provide palliation in patients with advanced disease in whom previous myelosuppressive treatment or advanced age precludes combination chemotherapy.[23]

Prognosis

Prognosis is determined primarily by the anatomic extent of disease as reflected in the pathologic state, the histopathologic type, the presence or absence of B symptoms, and age. It appears that differences in survival among stages I, II, and III are lessening. Currently, only stage IV shows a notably less favorable prognosis. In stages II and III, patients with B symptoms have a 10 percent poorer survival rate, and the prognosis becomes worse for patients 50 years of age and older.[31]

A definitive cure (normal life expectancy for the patient's age 10 or more years after treatment) is possible in 60 to 90 percent of patients with localized HD following early and intensive radiation therapy.[26]

In a study of patients with advanced HD treated with MOPP, 88 percent of whom had B symptoms while the other 12 percent did not, the survival rate was 64 percent among the complete responders, while 54 percent of all treated patients remained free of disease at 20 years follow-up. All the A patients achieved a CR, with 96 percent of the stage IIIA and 91 percent of stage IVA remaining relapse-free.[26]

Once a patient has maintained a CR for 4 years, the chance of relapse is less than 10 percent; the first 4 years of follow-up are when 90 percent of the relapses in HD will occur.[26]

NON-HODGKIN'S LYMPHOMA
Incidence and Etiology

The non-Hodgkin's lymphomas (NHL) represent a wide-ranging subgroup of lymphoid tumors. Approximately 15,000 new cases occur annually in the United States; about 13,200 deaths are due to NHL each year. Around 25 percent of NHL cases develop between 50 and 59 years of age, and the peak risk is at 60 to 69 years. NHL occurs in males at an only slightly higher rate (1.4 : 1) than in females.[23]

As with IID, the cause of NIIL is unknown. A viral cause has been suggested for some of the lymphomas. This theory stems from the implication of the Epstein-Barr virus in Burkitt's lymphoma, but there is no proof of a causal relationship. Chronic immunosuppressive therapy in organ transplant recipients has recently been associated with lymphocytic and histiocytic malignancies.[32] Other immunodeficiency syndromes are associated with an increased incidence of lymphomas. This has led to further speculation concerning either a viral etiology or an induced immunologic deficit allowing proliferation of a malignant clone.[23]

Classification

Histologic classification of NHL has recently become more standardized by the development of the Working Formulation of NHL for Clinical Usage, which resulted from a study by the National Cancer Institute to provide a link between the six main classification systems previously in use. However, it has proved to be more than a link between the earlier systems and has become widely used on its own in modern clinical studies.[33] An outline of this system is presented in Table 5-4.

Staging

The anatomic staging system used is the same as for HD. Staging laparotomy is generally not indicated for patients with NHL, most of whom are elderly, as it rarely affects treatment procedures. The exception is its use to rule out systemic disease in those patients who appear to have localized disease (especially younger patients), in whom radiation treatment is intended to encompass all disease with the goal of cure.[23,33]

Clinical Features

Signs and symptoms are similar to those of HD. Differences include a greater propensity for early involvement of oropharyngeal lymphoid tissue, skin, gastrointestinal tract, and bone and a much higher rate of bone marrow

Table 5-4. National Cancer Institute Working Formulation for Non-Hodgkin's Lymphomas

Low-grade malignancy
  A Malignant lymphoma, small lymphocytic
  B Malignant lymphoma, follicular. Predominantly small cleaved cell
  C Malignant lymphoma, follicular. Mixed small cleaved and large cell

Intermediate-grade malignancy
  D Malignant lymphoma, follicular. Predominantly large-cell
  E Malignant lymphoma, diffuse. Small cleaved cell
  F Malignant lymphoma, diffuse. Mixed small- and large-cell
  G Malignant lymphoma, diffuse. Large-cell

High-grade malignancy
  H Malignant lymphoma. Large-cell, immunoblastic
  I Malignant lymphoma. Lymphoblastic
  J Malignant lymphoma. Small noncleaved (including Burkitt's lymphoma)

Miscellaneous
  Composite   Extramedullary plasmacytoma
  Mycosis fungoides   Unclassifiable
  Histiocytic   Other

(From Mead and Whitehouse,[33] with permission.)

involvement. Gastrointestinal primaries occur fairly often in children with NHL (over one-third) as opposed to HD. Transformation to lymphoma occurs in about 13 percent of lymphocytic leukemia cases.[23]

Treatment and Prognosis

Low-Grade Lymphoma

Low-grade lymphoma accounts for 40 percent of NHL cases. It presents as enlarged lymph nodes, which often wax and wane in size; usually occurs in middle to late age; and commonly has a long, indolent clinical course. Extranodal sites of presentation are rare; bone marrow infiltration is common.

Radiation therapy is the treatment of choice for stage I and often for stage II disease. Advanced-stage patients without bulky disease or symptoms may be managed by simply watching and treating, as necessary, with single alkylating agents. Intensive chemotherapy alone or in combination with radiation therapy does not provide any better outcome than this method of treatment.[33] Median survival is usually 7 to 10 years.[33]

Intermediate-Grade Lymphoma

Intermediate-grade lymphoma accounts for 40 to 45 percent of NHL cases. Primary presentation may occur at almost any site, and it may evolve from a known low-grade lymphoma. Treatment will be described in terms of the management of nodal-based diffuse large cell lymphoma, which is the most common subtype in this category.

In stage I treatment is somewhat controversial. Radiation therapy alone has been reported to be highly successful in certain selected patients. Chemotherapy alone has also been successful in stage I patients. Chemotherapy is the treatment of choice for disease in stages II to IV, as disease in these stages is highly sensitive to chemotherapy. Regimens devised in the early to mid 1970s, such as C-MOPP and Cytoxan-hydroxydaunorubicin-Oncovin-prednisone (CHOP) (see Table 5-3) achieved a CR in about 60 percent of cases and long-term disease-free survival in 33 percent. Newer regimens such as methotrexate-bleomycin-Adriamycin-Cytoxan-Oncovin-dexamethasone (M-BACOD), methotrexate-Adriamycin-Cytoxan-Oncovin-prednisone-bleomycin (MACOP-B), and prednisone–VP-16–methotrexate-Adriamycin-Cytoxan followed by MOPP (ProMACE-MOPP) (Table 5-3) have CR rates of over 80 percent, and long-term survivors number at 60 to 70 percent.[26,33]

High-Grade Lymphoma

High-grade lymphoma represents 15 to 20 percent of NHL cases. These neoplasms are among the most rapidly growing known in humans. Lymphoblastic lymphoma, which most frequently presents as a mediastinal mass and most often occurs in young men, will spread early on to the bone marrow and the CNS. Burkitt's lymphoma is also highly aggressive and has a propensity to metastasize to the CNS. Immediate and intensive combination chemotherapy is always used for treatment, along with intrathecal chemotherapy for CNS prophylaxis. Approximately 40 to 45 percent of those with lymphoblastic lymphoma may achieve a cure; the cure rate in Burkitt's lymphoma relates to stage of disease at presentation.[23,33] The relapse-free survival curve for NHL shows that most adverse events tend to occur in the first 2 years; fewer than 10 percent of patients relapse once a CR has been maintained for 2 years.[26]

Extranodal Lymphoma

Occasionally, lymphoma may present at an extranodal site, affecting almost any organ. The stomach, thyroid, skin, breast, brain, and testes are common sites for such a neoplasm. Staging is the same as for lymph node lymphoma. Treatment is by surgery (with or without radiation therapy) if the disease is confined to the site of presentation. Combination chemotherapy must always be used if the disease is disseminated.[23]

Bone Marrow Transplantation for NHL

For patients with NHL who relapse after induction remission, the prognosis is not good. In a study of 398 patients with recurrent NHL, only 11 patients (2.8 percent) could be identified who were alive in CR 2 years after treatment.

Recently, BMT has become another option for such patients. Those treated while in first relapse or second remission obtain the best results, showing a 2-year disease-free survival rate of 40 percent.[34]

MULTIPLE MYELOMA

Incidence and Etiology

The incidence of multiple myeloma in the U.S. is estimated at about 9,600 cases per year, fairly equally distributed between males and females. The median age at diagnosis is 60, with over 90 percent of cases occurring after the age of 40; cases have occurred rarely in teenagers.[23,25] The cause is not known, but a possible etiology points to an inappropriate response to an initial antigenic stimulus.[23]

Clinical Features and Complications

Multiple myeloma is a lymphoproliferative disorder associated with plasma cells; bone and bone marrow are the main sites of involvement. Plasma cells are the most mature form of activated B lymphocytes and are responsible for the synthesis of the five major classes of immunoglobulins. In multiple myeloma, however, the proliferating plasma cells produce homologous immunoglobulin. High plasma concentrations of these homologous molecules inhibit normal synthesis of the other immunoglobulins.[23,30]

The pathophysiology of multiple myeloma is related partly to the autonomous proliferation of plasma cells and partly to the excessive production of immunoglobulin molecules. Painful osteolytic skeletal lesions may occur secondary to localized proliferation of malignant plasma cells in the bone marrow and bone. Proliferating plasma cells are believed to produce a protein called *osteoclast activating factor*, which stimulates resorption of bone.[8] Because of the osteolytic destruction of the bones, pathologic fractures are common. Simple maneuvers such as pushing up from a chair, turning in bed, coughing, or sneezing can cause arm or rib fractures. Spinal cord compression fractures can produce radicular or pleurisy-like pain, and peripheral neuropathy or cord compression can occur when nerves or spinal cord become impinged. Bone destruction causes mobilization of calcium into the bloodstream. The resultant hypercalcemia may be manifested by symptoms of weakness, nausea, and obtundation.[23,25,30]

Other secondary complications include pneumonia, urinary tract infection, and bacteremia. These occur primarily as a result of the inhibition of normal immunoglobulin synthesis, which causes deficient antibody production. Infection is also caused by leukopenia secondary to marrow replacement or to chemotherapy.[23,25,30]

Serum viscosity may be increased owing to the excessive levels of globulin protein. This results in fatigue, headache, somnolence, irritability, and visual disturbances. The hyperviscosity syndrome may induce anginal symptoms or congestive heart failure from the expansion in blood volume.[23,25,30]

An abnormal protein coating or thrombocytopenia may interfere with coagulation factors and cause a tendency toward abnormal bleeding. Rarely, the protein aggregate may act as a cryoglobulin, which precipitates in cold temperatures and causes Raynaud's phenomenon. Occasionally, carpal tunnel syndrome may occur as a result of amyloid deposits in tissue. Renal failure due to various factors may also be a complication.[23,25,30]

Antineoplastic Treatment

Radiation Therapy

A plasmacytoma (solitary area of plasma cell tumor) is treated with intensive local irradiation for possible cure. There is a tendency in such cases for disseminated myeloma to occur later, which may require several months of chemotherapy following irradiation. Palliative irradiation may be given to localized bone lesions for pain relief. Hemibody irradiation may be used in advanced refractory myeloma to alleviate widespread bone pain. In this technique delivery of 500 to 600 rads to the upper half of the body is followed by a similar dose to the lower body 6 to 8 weeks later. The toxicity of the large single dose may be avoided by fractionated hemibody irradiation.[23,25]

Chemotherapy

Alkylating agents, alone or with prednisone, are the drugs of choice in multiple myeloma. Maintenance therapy after initial induction of clinical remission (which represents only a fraction of reduction in the tumor burden) is of no further benefit.[23,25]

Prognosis

Median survival is 2 years from onset of therapy.[23]

MYCOSIS FUNGOIDES

Mycosis fungoides is a malignant lymphoma, which represents cancer of the thymus-derived T lymphocytes. It is a rare disease, and its natural history is not well understood. The disease appears to arise from or migrate to the skin and is characterized by multiple small, red scaling patches, plaque formation, or frank tumors. Studies at autopsy have shown that mycosis fungoides involves the lymph nodes, visceral organs, and CNS in 75, 50, and 14 percent of patients, respectively. The cells that characterize the disease (Sézary cells) are found in numerous benign cutaneous dermatoses that regress spontaneously, such as insect bites, eczema, and psoriasis. The earliest stages of mycosis fungoides may precede tumor development by 15 or more years. In early stages of the disease, localized treatment for extensive skin lesions has included total skin irradiation or topical application of nitrogen mustard. Widespread disseminated disease is treated with conventional chemotherapy.[30,35,36]

COMPLICATIONS OF LYMPHOMA AND/OR ITS TREATMENT

Infections such as bacterial septicemia, fungal infections, and herpes zoster are the most common complications of lymphoma treatment and are due to the leukopenia and immunosuppression resulting from therapy and/or the disease. Nausea, vomiting, and moderate to severe bone marrow suppression are common side effects of chemotherapy treatment with MOPP. MOPP may also cause aspermia and induction of early menopause.[23]

Irradiation treatment will cause hematologic depression in most patients, as well as possible skin changes, nausea, and vomiting. Infrequently, radiation pneumonitis, pericarditis, or clinical hypothyroidism is a problem. Joint fibrosis may occur on occasion. Even when appropriate shielding is used, the gonads still receive significant amounts of radiation when the pelvis is treated. Although common, azoospermia or menstrual dysfunction is usually temporary.[23] Genetic damage to germ cells has not been documented under these conditions. Combined-modality treatment may enhance some of the preceding complications.[23]

Another complication, which is becoming more recognized as the number of long-term survivors of HD and NHL increases, is avascular necrosis of the femoral and humeral heads. Among the protocol patients in continuous CR in a 1981 study, the incidence of avascular necrosis was 10.5 percent at 10 years.[35] More than one joint was usually involved, and the chief symptom was pain on movement or weight bearing. The onset of symptoms occurred from 6 to 78 months (mean 28 months) after the start of chemotherapy. Prednisone, one of the drugs used in combination chemotherapy treatment for HD and NHL, is believed to play a role in development of avascular necrosis. However, it is suspected that the drug combination used actually potentiates the prednisone because the dosage that these patients receive is much lower than the amounts demonstrated to cause bone necrosis in patients who received steroids in conjunction with organ transplants. The effect of radiation therapy on development of avascular necrosis also is not clear. In lymphoma patients receiving radiation treatment only, no cases of avascular necrosis have been reported. While some patients in these reports received only chemotherapy and no radiation therapy, it has been questioned whether radiation therapy, especially in full doses, may also be a potentiating element for bone necrosis.[35]

Although avascular necrosis may cause considerable morbidity, another even more serious long-term sequela is development of a second malignancy. Approximately 5 percent of patients successfully treated with combined-modality therapy for advanced HD develop acute leukemia. Undifferentiated NHL may occur in 2 to 5 percent of treated HD patients.[35]

Complications secondary to progressive lymphoma may include various cardiopulmonary and neurologic problems. Neurologic deficits can be a result of meningeal carcinomatosis. When malignant cells are deposited within the lepto-meninges, symptoms may include weakness, headache, diplopia, or other cranial nerve root signs. Spinal cord compression can occur secondary to growth of lymphoma through the intervertebral foramina into the epidural space from adjacent prevertebral lymph nodes. This will cause pain, progressive weakness, and sensory loss.

Superior vena cava syndrome in patients with lymphoma may occur as a result of extrinsic pressure by enlarged lymph nodes. Clinical features include facial edema; dilated veins in the scalp, chest wall, and neck; and dyspnea or orthopnea. These symptoms are usually effectively relieved by radiation treatment.[30] Pericardial effusion and tamponade can occur in the lymphoma patient as a result of tumor extension or diffuse thickening with constrictive pericarditis. Tachycardia and dyspnea are secondary to the resultant decrease in cardiac output plus systemic venous congestion. Diagnosis and treatment are both accomplished by pericardiocentesis.[30] Malignant pleural effusion is another complication that also produces dyspnea. Thoracocentesis may provide relief.[30]

Complications secondary to multiple myeloma have been previously addressed in that section. General debility and poor physical conditioning may result in any patient who has had to endure some of the above complications.

PHYSICAL THERAPY INTERVENTION

In light of the preceding list of possible complications, it is easy to see the need for physical therapy intervention in patients with lymphoma. Although a large proportion of these patients are able to achieve long-term, disease-free survival with relatively little to no lasting morbidity in the process, those who are not so fortunate may have to contend with a number of disease- and/or treatment-related complications. Generally, physical therapy is provided to these patients in the same manner and with the same rationale as to patients with similar problems unrelated to cancer. It is important, though, to be fully cognizant of the underlying diagnosis, the medical treatment rendered, and what the current or possible future complications of both may be. These factors may affect the physical therapy program for the individual patient.

One should be aware on a daily basis of the platelet count, the hematocrit and hemoglobin values, and the white blood cell count, which when low can respectively cause increased risk of bleeding, increased cardiopulmonary stress, and infection/high fever. General hematologic guidelines proposed by Dietz in 1979 specify no exercise if hematocrit is below 25 percent, hemoglobin below 8 mg/dl, platelets below 20,000/mm^3, or white blood cells below 500/mm^3 with fever. Resisted exercise should not be used when platelet count drops below 50,000/mm^3, and the exercise should be mild when hemoglobin is decreased to 8 to 10 mg/dl.[37]

In patients with lytic bone lesions, it is necessary to confer with the physician regarding the stability and weight-bearing potential of the limb, to avoid resistive exercise to the affected limb, and to instruct or assist in functional mobility so as not to stress the weakened bone(s). Pain may precede radiologic changes of osteolytic destruction, as up to 50 percent of bone mass must be lost before a lesion becomes apparent radiographically. Bone demineralization and osteoporosis are enhanced by immobility; thus it is very important that the patient maintain as high a level of activity as possible. This may be facilitated by use of ambulatory aids. Also, bracing may help to unload and/or restrict movement in the spine and thereby reduce pain.

The patient with complications from lymphoma and/or its treatment may be very debilitated as a result of prolonged immobility. Such individuals will require a very carefully graded and monitored program of rehabilitation and most often cannot be "pushed" as can patients without the cancer diagnosis, as their reserves may be very depleted. Emotional support should be ongoing throughout all phases of the illness and disability. It is important to keep in mind the patient's goals, stage of disease, and general prognosis so as to appropriately direct physical therapy to the preventive, restorative, supportive, or palliative level.

REFERENCES

1. Lichtman MA, Segel GB: The leukemias, p. 370. In Rubin P (ed): Clinical Oncology. 6th ed, American Cancer Society, Atlanta, 1983
2. Jacobs AD, Gale RP: Recent advances in the biology and treatment of acute lymphoblastic leukemia in adults. N Engl J Med 311:1219, 1984
3. Weinberg KI, Seigel SE: Acute lymphoblastic leukemia. p. 25. In Gale RP (ed): Leukemia Therapy. Blackwell Scientific Publications, Boston, 1983
4. Robison LL, Nesbit ME: Treatment of acute leukemia in childhood. p. 1. In Wiernik PH (ed): Contemporaty Issues in Clinical Oncology: Leukemias and Lymphomas. Churchill Livingstone, New York, 1985
5. Champlin RE: Acute myelogenous leukemia. p. 99. In Gale RP (ed): Leukemia Therapy. Blackwell Scientific Publications, Boston, 1983
6. Jacobs AD, Gale RP: Acute lymphoblastic leukemia in adults. p. 71. In Gale RP (ed): Leukemia Therapy. Blackwell Scientific Publications, Boston, 1983
7. Gralnick HR: Recent advances in the classification and identification of prognostic factors in acute lymphoblastic leukemia. Intern Med Specialist, 3(11):108, 1982
8. Champlin RE: Chronic myelogenous leukemia. p. 147. In Gale RP (ed): Leukemia Therapy. Blackwell Scientific Publications, Boston, 1983
9. Foon KA, Gale RP: Chronic lymphocytic leukemia. p. 165. In Gale RP (ed): Leukemia Therapy. Blackwell Scientific Publications, Boston, 1983
10. Johns Hopkins Hospital: Nursing flow sheet protocol #8410 for induction of remission in patients with AML. Johns Hopkins Hospital, Baltimore
11. Marmont AM: Allogeneic bone marrow transplantation for chronic granulocytic leukemia: Progress and controversies. Acta Haematol (Basel) 78:suppl 1, 181–186, 1987
12. Johns Hopkins Hospital; Nursing flow sheet, protocol #8302 for Induction of remissions in patients with ALL. Johns Hopkins Hospital, Baltimore
13. Yee GC, McGuire TR: Allogeneic bone marrow transplantation in the treatment of hematologic diseases. Clin Pharm 4:149, 1985
14. Jansen J, Provisor AJ, Vaughan J, et al: Interstitial pneumonitis after bone marrow transplantation: From last resort to preferred therapy. Indian Med 265, 1985
15. Santos GW, Saral R, Burns WH, et al: Allogeneic, syngeneic and autologous marrow

transplantation in the acute leukemias and lymphomas—Baltimore experiences. Acta Haematol (Basel) 78:suppl. 1, 175–180, 1987

16. Holtzman LS: Physical therapy intervention following bone marrow transplantaion. Clin Management, 8(2): 1988
17. Weiner RS, Bortin MM, Gale RP, et al: Interstitial pneumonitis after bone marrow transplantation. Ann Intern Med 104:168, 1986
18. Prentice HG, Brenner MK: Bone marrow transplantation in acute or chronic leukemia. Acta Haematol (Basel) 78:suppl. 1, 194–197, 1987
19. Applebaum FR, Fisher LD, Thomas ED: Chemotherapy v. marrow transplantation for adults with acute non-lymphocytic leukemia: A five year follow-up. Blood, 72:178, 1988
20. Hafliger B, Gratwohl A, Tichelli A, et al. High-dose ara-C and VP-16 before conditioning for bone marrow transplantation in patients with high-risk leukemia. Semin Oncol, 14(2):suppl. 1, 134–138, 1987
21. Herzig RH, Coccia PF, Strandjord SE, et al: Bone marrow transplantation for acute leukemia and lymphoma with high dose cytosine arabinoside and total body irradiation. Semin Oncol 14(2):suppl. 1, 139–140, 1987
22. Gribben JG, Vaughan HB, Linch DC: The potential value of very intensive therapy with autologous bone marrow rescue in the treatment of malignant lymphomas. Hematol Oncol, 5(4):281, 1987
23. Bakemeier RF, Zagars G, Cooper R, Rubin P: The malignant lymphomas. p. 346. In Rubin P (ed): Clinical Oncology for Medical Students and Physicians—A Multidisciplinary Approach. American Cancer Society, Atlanta, 1983
24. Walter JB: An Introduction to the Principles of Disease. WB Saunders, Philadelphia, 1977
25. Baldy, CM: Hematologic disorders, p. 184. In Carroll DP, Boynton SD, Cowell MW (eds): Pathophysiology. McGraw-Hill, New York, 1982
26. DeVita VT, Hubbard SM, Longo DL: The chemotherapy of lymphomas: Looking back, moving forward. Cancer Res 47:5810, 1987
27. Freireich EJ, Keating M, Cabnillas F, Barlogie B: The hematologic malignancies. Cancer 54:2741, 1984
28. Vianna NJ: Evidence for infectious component of Hodgkin's disease and related considerations. Cancer Res 36:663, 1976
29. Konrad PN, Erti JE: Hodgkin's disease. p. 39. In Pediatric Oncology. Medical Examination Publishing Co., New York, 1978
30. Skarin A, Canellos G, Mauch P, Neiman R: Lymphoma. p. 291. In Cady B (ed): Cancer Manual. American Cancer Society, Massachusetts Div., Boston, 1986
31. Kaplan HS: Hodgkin's disease: Unfolding concepts concerning its nature, management, and prognosis. Cancer 45:2439, 1980
32. Penn, I: The incidence of malignancies in transplant recipients. Transplant Proc 7:323, 1975
33. Mead GM, Whitehouse JM: Modern management of non-Hodgkin's lymphoma. Br Med J 293:577, 1986
34. Applebaum FR, Thomas ED: Bone marrow transplantation for malignant lymphoma. Eur J Cancer Clin Oncol 23:263, 1987
35. Prosnitz LR, Lawson JP, Friedlander GE, et al: Avascular necrosis of bone in Hodgkin's disease patients treated with combined modality therapy. Cancer 47:2793, 1981
36. Hallahan D, Griem M, Griem S, et al: Mycosis fungoides involving the central nervous system. J Clin Oncol 4:1638, 1986
37. Pfalzer C: Aerobic exercise for patients with disseminated cancer. Clin Man Phys Ther 8(2):28, 1988

6 | Rehabilitation of the Sarcoma Patient

Marsha H. Lampert
Cheryl Gahagen

SOFT TISSUE SARCOMAS

Physical therapy has become an important partner to the management team working to improve the quality of life for patients diagnosed with soft tissue sarcoma. As recently as the early 1970s, the standard surgical treatment for a high-grade sarcoma was amputation at or above the next joint proximal to the tumor.

Recently, modern scanning devices have resulted in earlier diagnosis and conservative surgery, called limb-sparing (LS). The new diagnostic tools include computed tomography (CT), used to evaluate the extent of the disease by delineating the relationship of the tumor to major structures; magnetic resonance imaging (MRI), used to assess the proximity of tumors to joints and to distinguish between fat, muscle tendon, bone, and blood vessels; arteriography, used to determine blood flow; and bone scans, used to demonstrate inflammatory changes at bone margins. One cannot discount the relevance of conventional x-ray devices as well. Limb-sparing surgery requires a reliance on adjuvant treatments such as radiation therapy and chemotherapy to improve disease-free survival.

Soft tissue sarcomas are a group of malignant tumors arising in the extraskeletal soft connective tissues that support and surround almost all other anatomic structures in the body. Approximately 30 histologic types of sarcomas have been identified, which have a common embryologic history, originating from the same primitive mesodermal layer. They are named after the cell of origin (e.g., synovial cell sarcoma from tendon, liposarcoma from adipose tis-

111

sue, neurofibrosarcoma from neural sheaths). All these are similar in pathologic appearance, clinical presentation and behavior. Histology does not seem to have an impact on prognosis.[1]

Approximately 4,500 new cases of soft tissue sarcoma are diagnosed in the United States annually, representing less than 1 percent of all cancers. These cases result in 1,000 deaths each year and an overall survival rate of 70 to 80 percent. There is no apparent sex or racial preference and no genetic predisposition. Sarcomas rank fifth of all cancers in children, occurring most often in the lower extremity (60 percent).[1] Head, neck, and trunk sarcomas rank second (24 percent), and 16 percent occur in the upper extremity.[2]

The site of the tumor can influence resectability and local control.[3] For the extremities the implication is that the more proximal the lesion, the less curable the disease. These lesions grow radially and compress the surrounding soft tissue as they enlarge. The reactive zone of tissue around the tumor, termed the *pseudocapsule*, is a permeable membrane, which allows microscopic cells to escape and ultimately spread the disease. The tumor extends longitudinally and invades along fascial planes, nerves, and blood vessels. It rarely invades bone, although there may be an associated periosteal reaction. Rarely do the microscopic cells metastasize to lymph nodes

The tumor usually presents as an asymptomatic mass. The patient may have pain, swelling, or limitation of motion due to pressure or traction of the sarcoma on adjacent structures. Injuries can call attention to preexisting tumors, but no proven causal relationship has been identified to date.

DIAGNOSIS AND TREATMENT

The patient is typically referred to the cancer center following diagnosis by biopsy. Biopsy incisions are usually placed in a vertical line to the underlying muscle. An *incisional biopsy*, described as the removal of a small piece of tissue cut directly from the tumor, is made primarily for diagnostic purposes. *Excisional biopsy* involves removal of the tumor en bloc but leaves the capsule and microscopic cells behind. This has not been judged adequate treatment for soft tissue sarcoma.[2]

Following diagnosis by biopsy and appropriate screening by scans, staging of the disease takes place. This process determines the aggressiveness of the sarcoma and is necessary for appropriate treatment planning. The criteria for staging of soft tissue sarcoma are not well defined or universally accepted. Categories considered important include histologic type, frequency of mitotic figures in the specimen, degree of necrosis,[4] cellularity, vascularity, size of tumor, and metastatic potential, as well as the presence of local and distant metastases.

The American Joint Committee on Cancer and the Musculoskeletal Tumor Society for Bone and Soft Tissue Sarcomas state that the goal of staging is to determine the prognostic factors describing the risks of local recurrence and distant metastases, as well as the specific guidelines for surgical management and adjuvant therapies that are implied by these factors.

Enneking has described a system based on the interrelationship of grade (G); biologic aggressiveness; anatomic sites of the tumor (T), whether it is intra- or extracompartmental; and metastasis (M) to distant organs or lymph nodes. Subcutaneous tumors involving the skin have no longitudinal boundaries, and the deep fascia acts as a barrier to another tissue plane.[5]

Current trends in the selection of the most appropriate staging process support the concept that the higher the grade and the less differentiated the cell, the smaller the probability of disease-free interval and the lower the survival rates for high-grade sarcomas.

Metastasis may occur as a result of seeding when microscopic cells break off from the gross tumor mass and circulate in the blood. Tumor spillage may also occur during surgery, causing local or distant spread. Chemotherapy, used as an adjuvant to surgery, is most effective in treatment of microscopic disease.[6] The lungs are usually the most common site for metastasis with liver, bones, and brain the next most likely areas.

Treatment approaches for soft tissue sarcoma vary among facilities. Currently, several clinical trials are being conducted to determine how surgery, radiation therapy, and chemotherapy can best increase survival. The quality of that survival requires implementation of vigorous rehabilitation techniques in order to maximize function. The goals of physical therapy must include quality of survival with minimal life-style changes during treatment and for the future.[7]

Multiagent chemotherapy has become recognized as a necessary adjuvant to surgery. Various drugs have been used; soft tissue sarcoma cells not affected by one drug may be destroyed by another. Certain drugs disrupt the ability of both normal and cancer cells to grow and multiply. Chemotherapy programs include preoperative and/or postoperative courses of treatment. The length and frequency of the course may be modified by the medical oncologist, the policies of the facility, and/or the progressive changes in the stage of the disease.

Chemotherapy is given as a systemic treatment following wide excision and often in conjunction with radiation to destroy circulating sarcoma cells. Drugs of choice include vincristine, methotrexate, Adriamycin, Cytoxan, and actinomycin D. These may be administered intravenously, intramuscularly, orally, or by intra-arterial perfusion.

Regional treatment or local perfusion with Adriamycin[8,9] is accomplished with an indwelling arterial line placed in a major artery supplying the affected limb (e.g., the femoral artery in the lower extremity). This is done preoperatively to allow large tumors to regress, thus enabling surgeons to attempt conservative limb-sparing procedures and is coordinated with radiation therapy. Surgery is performed approximately 3 weeks later. Major complications that may result include infection, for which amputation would be the surgical treatment of choice. There may also be a problem of skin slough, causing further delay prior to the limb-sparing procedure.

The current philosophy of preoperative chemotherapy suggests that tumor margins may be more clearly delineated by necrosis of the peripheral cells, thus allowing a limb-sparing procedure. Circulating microscopic cells may also be destroyed or rendered sterile. At the time of surgery following preoperative chemotherapy, the pathologist is able to evaluate the effects of the chemotherapy on the tumor after it has been resected.

Postoperative chemotherapy is also a popular regimen. It is administered as soon as the surgical wound is healed. If there are complications as a result of surgery, chemotherapy will have to be delayed.

Side effects related to these protocols may include one, all, or several of the following: nausea, vomiting, alopecia, cardiomyopathy, peripheral (mixed sensorimotor) neuropathy, mucositis, myelosuppression, delayed healing, decreased endurance, amenorrhea, and sexual dysfunction.[10,11] Almost all these effects are reversible over time.

Additional experimental therapies are being explored in the laboratory setting, but as yet none has served the soft tissue sarcoma patient well. *Immunotherapy* uses substances produced by the body's own immune system (antibodies) to promote tumor destruction. These antibodies are activated or enhanced with biologic response modifiers (BRM) from the cells of the tumor removed from the patient. These cells are reinfused into the patient after the lymphocytes have been treated in the laboratory. Common names for these substances are *interleukin* and *interferon*.

Radiation therapy using a high-energy external beam is effective in sterilizing the area where the tumor is seated or from which the tumor has been excised. It is presumed to be an excellent adjuvant treatment for achieving local tumor control. The procedure involves placing a patient in a simulator in order to determine accurately the area to be radiated. A computer projects radiation beams to display a graphic contour of the patient. The site of the incision (for biopsy or excision), drainage holes if present, and a margin of 10 cm around the mass are generally included in the radiation field.

The decision to administer preoperative radiation can be made at staging. Radiation doses of 5,000 to 6,000 rads at 200 rads/day for 5 to 6 weeks are used to inactivate soft tissue sarcoma cells by as much as 99 percent,[12] thereby diminishing the possibility of distant seeding.[13] This process is used to kill peripheral cells in the tumor. Preoperative treatment my decrease the extent of surgery, thus also decreasing functional or cosmetic problems. Complications of preoperative radiation include predisposition of the long bones to fracture, as a result of devascularization, and delayed healing of the incision.[14]

If postoperative radiation therapy is required, a larger field is used to include all tissues involved at surgery. The use of shrinking field radiation minimizes skin sensitivity to this treatment. Shrinking fields limit the highest dose of radiation to the area of greatest possibility of recurrence. Surgical clips placed intraoperatively at the periphery of the excision define the involved area. A strip of normal tissue with half the cross-sectional area of the limb must be left untreated to ensure lymphatic drainage.[1] Initial treatments totaling 4,500 rads encompass all probable areas of local spread; the field is then reduced to the tumor bed for another 1,500 rads.

The advantages of postoperative treatment are that the histology can be confirmed and there can be efficient planning of fields.[13] The disadvantages include the creation by surgery of anaerobic areas, which decrease the blood and oxygen supply to the tumor bed, making it more resistant to radiation therapy. Radiation sensitizers may be used to correct this and are available in the form of drugs, hyperbaric oxygen chambers, or transfusions to correct anemia. Less popular is *brachytherapy*, in which radioactive (iridium 192) seeds[9] are temporarily implanted into the tumor bed. This procedure is used for anatomic areas difficult to treat by external beam radiation. Hyperthermia may also increase the effect of radiation to the area. The part to be radiated is heated to 42 to 45°C through a controlled temperature rise. In rehabilitation, thermal modalities are not used immediately before or after the radiation treatment because of the difficulty in ascertaining skin and cell temperature, which is necessary to ensure accurate radiation dose delivery.

The patient must always be placed in an exact and reproducible position for radiation therapy, which may be accomplished by using casts to duplicate the posture each day. The position must be as comfortable as possible. Wedges may be used to block or avoid radiation "splatter" to sensitive areas such as the spinal cord.

Mild radiation reactions, such as dermatitis or erythema, are expected. Severe responses include fibrosis of connective tissue, resulting in a contracture when the total joint has been irradiated.

Additional acute changes can occur during treatment, usually involving the rapidly proliferating cells of hair or skin. There may be burns to the area and open wounds requiring whirlpool treatment and debridement. Radiation is often temporarily discontinued if the reactions are severe. Physical therapy should be carefully monitored during this time so as to minimize or prevent these self-limiting problems through an active exercise program. Direct supervision may not be necessary, but education of the patient regarding these changes is paramount.

Intermediate changes can occur up to 6 months following cessation of treatment. Increasing fibrosis within muscle tissue can occur, promoting contractures, which may be reversible with active stretching. Chronic changes occurring in supportive tissues may be irreversible despite physical therapy. Bone necrosis, endarteritis and decreased elasticity of lymphatic channels can cause severe edema, pain, and decreased function.[7] Cellular and vascular necrosis may lead to bone fracture, which is slow to heal owing to diminished blood supply.

Intracompartmental tumors arise within a muscle group and do not involve bone or essential neurovascular structures. Limb-sparing surgery is a reasonable option for these cases. An *extracompartmental* tumor originates between muscle groups or involves more than a single group. These lesions may involve bone or neurovascular elements. Historically, amputations have been the treatment of choice, but limb sparing is now an option. Through limb sparing, the surgeon attempts to preserve as much function as possible without compromise of survival.

The criteria for wide local excision or limb sparing are that either the tumor must be totally resectable, without significant involvement or dissection of major vessels and nerves or reconstruction utilizing bone grafts, or else an endoprosthesis must provide limb function equal or superior to the function of a prosthesis. It should be remembered that a limb-sparing procedure is more complex than amputation. The duration of surgery is longer, and infection and pain may be more common and physical therapy more intense.[7] The presumed psychological advantage of limb sparing versus amputation has yet to be established.[15,16]

Authorities agree that rehabilitation should begin at the time of diagnosis, prior to surgical intervention, and should continue for the rest of the patient's life. Planning and implementing effective physical therapy are accomplished through understanding of the course of the disease as well as the outcomes associated with particular treatments. Educated patients can alter the impact of their disease and treatments with positive thinking and less anxiety. Physical therapy planning should be included in the initial staging, physical examination, and orientation of the patient.[17] With patients' permission, all teaching should include their personal support systems.

Assistive devices should be made available in hospital rooms to encourage early independence. These items include over-the-bed trapezes for bed mobility, seat cushions in wheelchairs, and grab bars in the bathrooms.

PHYSICAL THERAPY CONSIDERATIONS

It is not within the scope of this text to review all basic physical therapy procedures but owing to the uniqueness of some techniques, treatment recommendations for selected anatomic sites are in order. Functional limits in some cases are obvious and do not require discussion.

Partial or total scapulectomies are procedures performed when tumors involve the scapula or the surrounding soft tissue. Removal of all or part of the scapula, including the glenoid fossa, may be necessary. If the glenoid complex is left intact, upper extremity function may be close to normal. Removal of the glenoid creates restrictions of arm movement, often actively beyond 90 degrees, and pain and complaints of fatigue at the end of the day are not uncommon. Transcutaneous electrical nerve stimulation (TENS) and a sling for temporary support may be adequate for the individual to function normally.

Retroperitoneal tumors are often difficult to excise and often recur owing to the difficulty in attaining negative surgical margins. Physical therapy is usually requested in conjunction with the adjuvant radiation therapy. It is not unusual for the femoral nerve to be within the radiation field which requires protection and support of the muscles innervated by this nerve (see later section on quadriceps excision). Edema is a secondary complication if the inguinal nodes lie within the field. Use of support hose is recommended as well as education of patients to elevate their lower extremities throughout the day.

A buttock resection is performed when there is en bloc resection of the gluteus maximus. Care is exercised by the surgeon to avoid damaging the sciatic nerve intraoperatively. Closure of these wounds may be tenuous as a result of the removal of large tumors in this area. The patient may complain of difficulty in stair climbing, pain along the incision, and altered body image. Frequently, radiation will disrupt normal sexual functioning and bowel habits.

The physical therapist may encourage strengthening of other hip girdle muscles and provide seat cushions. A custom buttock may be fabricated out of thermoplastic material to resemble the contralateral buttock. This is secured to the undergarments with Velcro.

An internal hemipelvectomy[18] may be performed with a diagnosis of soft tissue sarcoma in the upper thigh and/or buttock or ilium. The sacrum is transected through the neural foramina, with resection of the hemipelvis, proximal femur, and occasionally the bladder, rectum, or genitalia. In cases of intrapelvic tumor, the peritoneal cavity will be entered. Stabilization of the pelvis and femur requires prolonged bed rest with skeletal traction to allow for fusion and maintenance of as much leg length as possible. Shoe lifts are imperative as soon as bed restrictions are removed, which is usually 3 to 6 weeks postsurgery. Partial weight bearing using crutches is allowed until total union of the remaining pelvis or ilium and femur occurs. This process may require up to 6 months. Strengthening of the distal muscles and upper extremities through repetitive active exercise against gravity is important. Sensation generally remains intact, with few complaints of pain. Variations of this procedure are common, and close cooperation between the therapist and surgeon is necessary to monitor progress.

The thigh is one of the most difficult areas in which to attain a high level of tumor control without significant morbidity, and historically it is an area most likely to develop a soft tissue sarcoma. Tumors are large when found and are masked by bulky muscle tissue. Sometimes, as a result of radiation splatter to the upper medial thigh, sexual dysfunction and chronic lymphedema may occur. Joint dysfunction and pain are not unusual symptoms but may be later findings.[7] For most wide local excisions of the thigh, there is prolonged serosanguinous drainage. When the drainage has decreased or tubing has been removed, ambulation and active exercises can begin in earnest.

The patient may be placed in splinting devices such as commercial knee immobilizers and posterior foot splints. These can be removed for supervised exercise and dressing changes. These appliances protect the part from poor positioning and prevent wounds from being inadvertently overstretched, particularly when the incision crosses a joint.

The definitive treatment of an extracompartmental soft tissue sarcoma within the anterior thigh requires total excision of the quadriceps muscle[19] (Fig. 6-1). The muscle is removed from origin to insertion in cases of high-grade tumors. Radiation is not recommended following this procedure as it would involve crossing two joint spaces. The patient remains at bed rest in a knee immobilizer until restrictions are lifted. Ankle motion should be encouraged. When ambulation is appropriate, partial weight bearing in the splint can be

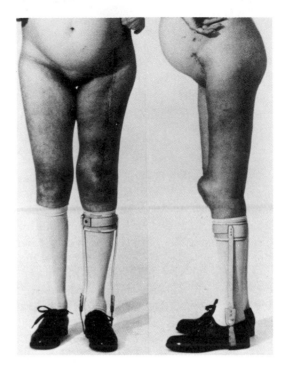

Fig. 6-1. Postoperative appearance following total quadriceps muscle excision. Deficit in thigh mass observed in lateral view (right). (From Sugarbaker and Nicholson,[45] with permission.)

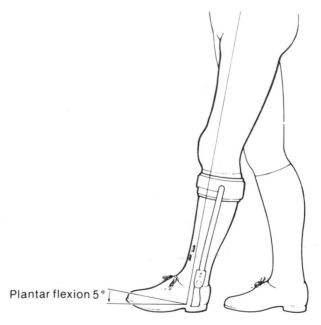

Plantar flexion 5°

Fig. 6-2. Ankle-foot orthosis for total quadriceps muscle excision permitting 5 degrees of plantar flexion and zero degrees from neutral dorsi-flexion. (From Sugarbaker and Nicholson,[45] with permission.)

allowed. At approximately 2 weeks, a dual-channel aluminum ankle-foot ortho-sis is provided, which blocks dorsiflexion and allows 5 degrees of plantar flexion (Fig. 6-2). An extension moment is created at the knee on heel strike with the ground reactive force anterior to the knee axis (TKA line), forcing the knee into extension.

Without the brace, the knee can extend by locking in hyperextension and increasing the lordotic curve of the lumbar spine. This is not acceptable for activity for the obvious biomechanical reasons. Falling and loss of balance as well as back pain are not unusual results of these postures.

Adductor group excisions are done for sarcomas of the medial thigh. Lymph nodes are not deliberately removed as in groin dissection, but because of their proximity may be sacrificed in the specimen. Edema is a common sequela of either the surgery or the radiation (Fig. 6-3).

Initially physical therapy of the involved extremity is kept at a minimum. Isometric contractions of the quadriceps appears to increase drainage volume. Support stockings, either custom or commercial, are recommended for all up-right activities. Rarely are there complaints of motor dysfunction with this procedure; however, complaints of pain and edema are common. Patients should be instructed to elevate their legs and educated regarding proper skin care. Women should be advised to take precautions during leg shaving.

Excision of the hamstring group occasions few problems. Common com-plaints are stiffness following prolonged sitting and unsteadiness when running. Chronic problems, noted long after treatments have been completed, include contractures at the knee and ankle. Stretching programs must be emphasized and continued, and women should be discouraged from wearing high heels. If the sciatic nerve is sacrificed, motor loss combined with leg anesthesia, will ensue, promoting a tendency for skin to ulcerate with trauma. An ankle-foot orthosis will be necessary to assist with foot clearance. Following initial treat-ments, an ankle fusion or a posterior tibialis transfer may be recommended. The patient must be educated as to proper foot care, shoes, and orthosis application.

Gastrocnemius muscle excision in the posterior compartment of the leg may require the addition of a properly placed rocker bottom on the sole of the shoe. Daily heel cord stretching is essential and should be encouraged.

Irradiation of the foot is a difficult procedure and is generally avoided if the sole of the foot or Achilles tendon is involved. This area is subject to trauma and skin breakdown. Custom inserts can be made to provide proper foot contact. If the posterior tibial nerve is excised, sensation is interrupted but no other func-tional problems are noted.

Wide local excisions of the upper extremity do not result in complications as severe as those seen in the lower extremity. However, it remains important to understand the procedures that are performed in order to instruct the patient about achieving maximum use of the extremity. The population followed most frequently by me (Lampert) has been patients who have undergone major nerve resections or limb salvage procedures. Tumors found in the upper extremity are generally smaller than those in the lower, allowing for more conservative sur-gery. Rarely are whole muscle groups involved. Tumors of the hand that require

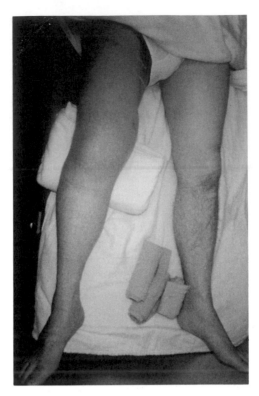

Fig. 6-3. Medial wall excision for adductor muscle group. Five days postoperatively edema can be observed throughout the right lower extremity.

radiation and major resections may render the hand insensate; for these, amputation options should be considered. Postoperatively, morbidity is less in the upper extremity than in the lower. Drainage is less prolonged, wound infection less frequent, and radiation therapy better tolerated.

The Tikhoff-Linberg procedure for tumors of the proximal humerus and scapula is one chosen in lieu of a forequarter amputation if there is no chest wall or neurovascular involvement. Function and support of the upper extremity are provided by multiple muscle transfers and skeletal reconstruction using a customized endoprosthesis to maintain arm length and to stabilize the remaining humerus.[20] (Fig. 6-4). Patients using this device incur a risk of infection and potential loosening of the prosthesis in the distal humerus. Hand and forearm functions are approximately normal, but there is no true shoulder motion. Passively, the joint can be moved to 90 degrees in flexion or abduction. There are no active rotations.

Pain and edema are minimal with this procedure except in the acute recovery phase. There have been isolated cases of transient nerve palsies following surgery. Generally patients are placed in a sling that prevents abduction (Vel-

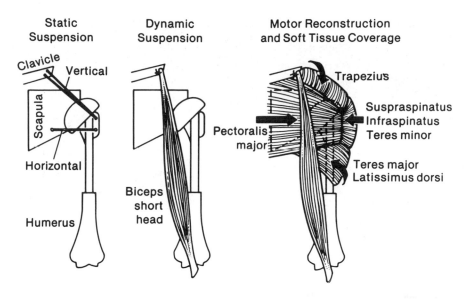

Fig. 6-4. Stages of intraoperative suspension and reconstruction for Tikhoff-Linberg procedure. (From Sugarbaker and Nicholson,[45] with permission.)

peau sling) postoperatively. Maceration of axillary skin is sometimes a problem, as the arm cannot be moved from the side. Active elbow flexion and extension within the sling are allowed. Approximately 3 weeks postoperatively, the sling is removed for full hand and elbow motion. Normal activities are encouraged, but weights exceeding 20 pounds should never be lifted because of undue traction on reconstructed muscles.

To ensure a positive body image, a commercial shoulder pad may be added to support a brassiere strap or heavy overcoat. A suggestion may be made to the female patient to purchase a jogging or sport brassiere for comfort.

Soft tissue sarcomas in the axilla may necessitate sacrifice of the long head of the triceps and the latissiumus dorsi as it nears the axilla. Lymphatic drainage following surgery is usually significant. If radiation is prescribed, placement of the patient in a salute position of at least 100 degrees flexion/abduction and 75 degrees external rotation is essential and needs to be accomplished as soon as possible. For spasm of the pectoral muscle, TENS may offer relief. Skin breakdown is not uncommon with radiation owing to perspiration in the axilla and may cause several interruptions in treatment. Use of deodorants or body creams is not allowed unless cleared by the radiologist. Wearing of cotton undershirts for absorbency is recommended. Range of motion at the shoulder should be maintained as long as there is adequate skin integrity.

The elbow is vulnerable to trauma when the radial nerve or head of the radius is excised. Emphasis is placed on maintaining finger and wrist range of motion in a functional posture (Fig. 6-5). Dynamic splinting may be prescribed.

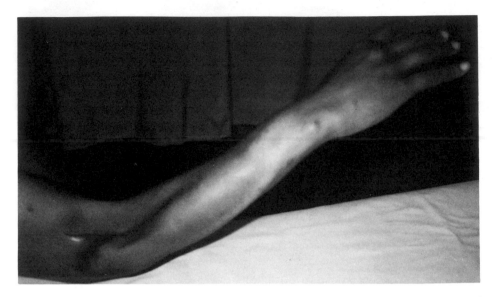

Fig. 6-5. One year following excision of radial nerve and head of radius with transfer of flexor carpi radialis for improved wrist and finger function.

If the wrist can be stabilized in some extension, the interossei and finger flexors may be utilized for prehension. The elbow should be protected by a padded cuff. Postsurgical tendon transfers using the flexor carpi radialis and thumb stabilizers may be attempted.

Like the foot, the hand is a difficult structure to radiate. It has an uneven surface allowing for variable differences in radiation absorption. Treatment has been accomplished successfully, but patient selection is very discriminating.

In summary, multiple problems can be expected as sequelae to treatments for soft tissue sarcoma. Osteoporosis or fractures may result from radiation therapy. Caution needs to be emphasized with patients involved in risk-taking situations. It is acceptable to swim, golf, and play tennis, but contact sports should be avoided. Edema due to inelasticity or excision of lymphatic channels is not uncommon. The therapist may suggest intermittent compression machines, support garments, and elevation of the limb. Pain may be concurrent with stiffness and edema. A trial of TENS may minimize the use of strong addictive analgesics, which in themselves modify quality of life. TENS allows patients to exert some control over treatment and recovery. Wound healing delays can invite infection in open areas. The patient must be instructed in proper skin care which may include light applications of vitamin E or aloe to the skin following completion of the course of radiation treatments. Deep massage may delay or prevent a hard, woody-appearing extremity. Deformity or defects can be remedied by fabricating cosmetic fillers from thermoplastic materials. Muscle fibrosis, resulting in contractures long after treatments have been concluded, is sometimes unavoidable.[21]

It is important to remember that many patients with soft tissue sarcomas are ideal candidates for physical therapy. There may be functional limitations as a direct result of their disease or as a result of the treatment. The barrier to optimal rehabilitation has been a failure in the past to identify these problems. The obligation of any rehabilitation service is to allow patients to achieve their fullest possible physical, psychological, social, vocational, and educational potentials.

PEDIATRIC SARCOMAS

The majority of pediatric bone and soft tissue sarcomas are highly malignant, rapidly growing, and predisseminated at diagnosis. Medical management must be aggressive, multimodal, and aimed at ablation of both primary and distant disease. Prior to the use of chemotherapy in the early 1970s, survival rate for pediatric sarcomas did not exceed 20 percent. The advent of multiagent chemotherapy regimens in combination with surgery and radiation therapy has increased survival rates two- to threefold. Through multi-institutional trials, cooperative study groups are establishing optimal treatments for various disease stages. As disease has been better defined through improved staging techniques and treatment protocols made more specific to the stage of disease, treatment morbidity has been lessened. Improving treatment efficacy permits new management options, such as limb salvage versus amputation, for disease control.

OSTEOSARCOMA

Osteosarcoma is the most common bone malignancy in children and is the second most common bone malignancy at all ages. The incidence of osteosarcoma is highest in the second decade of life, during which time 50 percent of cases are diagnosed.[22] Male incidence is almost double female incidence.

The etiology of osteosarcoma is unclear. The association of mitotically active metaphyseal cells with rapidly growing bones in a high-growth-rate population (taller adolescent boys) suggests that a high growth rate may predispose a bone site to neoplasia through accelerated mutation. The incidence of osteosarcoma is increased to 4 percent in previously irradiated bone and is increased in bone exposed to radium.[23] Adults with congenital bone disorders are genetically predisposed to osteosarcoma, as are children with bilateral retinoblastoma.

Osteosarcoma is a primary bone malignancy, characterized by osteoid production by malignant stroma cells. The tumor originates in the bone interior, penetrates through the cortex, spreads beneath the periosteum, and may invade soft tissue. It is generally located in the metaphyseal ends of long bones, presenting in the extremities in 75 percent of pediatric cases (femur 40 percent, tibia 16 percent, humerus 15 percent), with a lower incidence in the axial skeleton, clavicle, and scapula.[24] In adults the incidence of tumor in long bones and flat bones is equal.

Initial symptoms include sudden onset of pain and swelling at the tumor site. Decreased range of motion, erythema, and warmth are seen occasionally. Weakness, anemia, and weight loss are rare. Detectable metastatic disease may be present in up to 20 percent of cases at diagnosis, but micrometastases are suspected in all cases.[22] Tumor spreads hematogenously to lung and bone.

Diagnosis is usually made 3 months after onset of symptoms. As the doubling time for osteosarcoma is 20 to 38 days, treatment is radical and targets local and distant disease. Historically, primary tumor was eradicated by amputation above the proximal joint so as to eliminate suspected intramedullary tumor extension and skip lesions. Improved scanning has permitted transosseous amputation with 5- to 7-cm tumor-free margins. Local tumor control may be achieved with nonamputative limb salvage and internal prosthetic replacement in selected individuals.

Early limb salvage attempts were viewed as experimental as there was increased risk of local tumor recurrence.[5] This procedure was reserved for children near skeletal maturity who had small, noninvasive, distally located tumors. Original limb salvage complications included early and late infections, bone resorption, nerve palsies, and endoprosthetic problems, including stress fractures of the implant and loosening and penetration of the bone shaft by the implant.[26]

Local tumor recurrence rates are presently equal for amputation and limb salvage surgery.[27] Reconstructive procedures for restoration of osseous and joint continuity have varied and have included use of customized metallic endoprostheses, autoclaved autografts, and cadaver allografts. Endoprostheses are most common. Implant complications have been reduced by use of high-strength, lightweight alloys and methyl methacrylate fixation.[28]

Multiagent chemotherapy has significantly increased disease-free survival. The first agents found to be highly effective were Adriamycin and high-dose methotrexate. Encouraged by these results, Rosen and colleagues assessed tumor response in adjunctive trials of high-dose methotrexate, bleomycin, Cytoxan, and actinomycin D prior to surgical resection.[24] If tumor necrosis exceeded 80 percent, patients continued on the same protocol. If tumor necrosis was less than 80 percent, postoperative chemotherapy included Adriamycin and cisplatin. The preoperative screening of tumor response to chemotherapy appears to have significantly increased overall survival owing to the ability to select optimal individual chemotherapy.

Osteosarcoma is relatively radioresistant, with tumoricidal doses ranging from 70 to 120 gray (Gy). Radiation therapy may be used in conjunction with chemotherapy to treat unresectable skull, rib, or pelvic lesions and pulmonary and bone metastases.

The treatment outcome for recurrent disease has improved, partly because of the changing patterns of metastases. An increasing number of metastases are extrapulmonary and arise in distant bone; these are fewer in number and less malignant and present later in the clinical course.[29] Thus, the treatment outcome for metastatic disease is enhanced as these features may permit more extended and effective treatment.

The significant advances that have been made in the comprehensive management of osteosarcoma are reflected in the higher survival rates. The overall 5-year survival rate is 50 to 60 percent.[30]

Physical Therapy Intervention

Prior to the option of limb salvage, amputation was the treatment of choice for all patients with osteosarcoma of the extremity. If an en bloc resection with the required envelope of normal tissue demands sacrifice of major nerves, blood vessels, or muscle, amputation continues to be indicated. Surgeries are radical with wide tumor-free margins, resulting in high levels of amputation; 88 percent of all amputations are lower extremity, 50 percent are above the knee, and 27 percent are hip disarticulations or hemipelvectomies.[31] Because upper extremity amputations are less common, this chapter will address the lower extremity amputee.

The oncologic amputee faces multiple psychological and physical issues related to diagnosis of potentially terminal disease and long-term treatment.[32] In addition to losing a limb, the child encounters nausea and vomiting, alopecia, dropping blood counts with the possibility of decreased stamina, increased infections, and added hospitalizations. Anxiety, fear, pain, altered body image, and increased dependency are difficult issues for all patients, especially for the large proportion of patients who are adolescent and already making adjustments for psychosexual and physical development.

Physical therapy intervention begins preoperatively when the patient and family are educated regarding realistic capabilities and limitations of prosthetic function.[25] It should be explained that high-level amputations are consistent with high energy expenditure, precluding functional prosthetic use for some patients. Clarifying expectations and discussing the physical therapy program for residual limb conditioning and gait training preoperatively is the first step toward successful prosthetic training.

Instruction in bed mobility, transfer training, and ambulation and a residual limb conditioning program are initiated within a few days postoperatively. The patient participates in limb strengthening and range-of-motion exercises and is instructed in skin care and edema control via positioning and compressive wrapping using a stump shrinker or elastic bandage. The residual limb may be bandaged during surgery with a rigid dressing. As the dressing remains in place for several weeks, the risk of wound infection is minimized and postoperative edema is reduced. Gait training may be initiated within 1 week by attaching a pylon to the cast. The patient may be recast within 2 weeks for a temporary prosthesis worn for 1 to 2 months, which facilitates stump maturation and permits early gait training.

Recommendations for the prosthetic prescription are based on residual limb length and configuration, as well as on the patient's age, neuromuscular development, growth potential, and expected activity level. The goals of the patient and family are incorporated. Selection of componentry should be influenced by the fact that prosthetic replacement may be necessary in 1 to 2 years, depending on skeletal growth and the degree of mechanical wear caused by vigorous activities.

Once the needs of the patient are identified, a customized prosthesis is designed by selecting appropriate componentry. The advantages and disadvantages of every option must be weighed. This becomes evident with the initial choice between an exoskeletal and an endoskeletal system. The exoskeletal system is durable but heavy, and modifications are restricted to increasing limb length by placing wooden blocks between the foot and the shoe. The endoskeletal system is more cosmetic, lightweight, and modular (components can be easily adjusted, repaired, or replaced). This system is less durable and the foam cover often requires early replacement.

The essential ingredient for successful prosthetic fit is a suitable socket. Above-knee socket designs include the ischial weight-bearing, total contact, quadrilateral socket; the suction socket, which is built on a pressure gradient; and the narrow mediolateral socket. Midthigh levels are accommodated by the simpler, less expensive, quadrilateral socket, and limb volume changes are easily controlled by adjusting stump sock thickness as needed. When suspension becomes a problem with shorter limbs, a suction socket improves the limb-socket fit, but volume fluctuations affect fit significantly. Very short and bulbous limbs are best controlled in narrow mediolateral sockets because the proximal femur is well contained by the high lateral socket wall and tight mediolateral purchase. A neoprene pelvic belt encircling both the waist and the proximal socket is available as an auxiliary suspension system.

Prosthetic function is influenced by the selection of the prosthetic knee and foot. The most common and durable knee is the constant friction knee. A polycentric knee is preferred for higher levels, as the rotating axis enhances stability. The hydraulic knee best simulates normal walking because resistance changes with walking speed.

The standard prosthetic foot is the solid ankle–cushion heel (SACH) foot, designed with a soft heel to absorb shock. The solid ankle–flexible endoskeletal (SAFE) foot has mediolateral action and permits a smoother gait. Stored-energy (Seattle, carbon copy, Flex) feet are built with carbon fibers in a leaf spring design and return energy during the ground reaction phase. All feet are built to accommodate ¾-inch heels, and few, if any, accommodate heel height changes. Child sizes are not available in all prosthetic foot types.

Prosthetic gait training may be approached as instruction in the acquisition of a new gross motor skill, with the emphasis on achieving single-limb balance. The patient's pelvis must be balanced directly over the stance foot in order to avoid the common prosthetic gait deviations of ipsilateral trunk lean during prosthetic stance and a wide-based gait. Once good balance is achieved in single-limb standing and weight shifting, the level of the assistive device is reduced until the patient either reaches independent ambulation or is ambulating with a straight cane.

During this repetitive, tedious process, it is imperative to give the patient ongoing auditory and visual feedback. Patients should be encouraged to identify and correct deviations on their own as well. By progressing slowly with ample encouragement from the therapist, a near normal gait pattern is achieved. Gait deviations are not desirable for any amputee; this is particularly true for the pediatric amputee, as normal musculoskeletal stresses beginning at an early age can produce lifelong spine and joint problems. Gait training culminates when the child can ambulate on a community level, demonstrating good endurance without gait deterioration. Many children return to modified physical education and sports.

Reduction in residual limb volume may persist for a year or more postamputation, initially because of resolving edema followed by soft tissue atrophy. Volume fluctuations challenge fabrication and maintenance of fit of the prosthetic socket. In addition to changing stump sock thickness, the shrinking limb may be accommodated by using a temporary flexible socket with adjustable closures, by a series of flexible sockets in a rigid frame, or by modifying a permanent socket by filling it entirely or by padding specific areas. During this long period of stump maturation, the patient must comply with stump wrapping whenever the prosthesis is not used.

Chemotherapy may further complicate prosthetic gait training due to IV lines, nausea, and reduced stamina. Incisional healing and stump maturation may be delayed. If nausea results in decreased dietary intake with more than 5 percent body weight reduction, major socket reconstruction is usually necessary.

The physical therapist follows the patient to assess prosthetic fit and function as the child matures. A replacement prosthesis is indicated when the patient outgrows the socket or when the prosthesis can no longer be lengthened. Component options should be considered to meet the changing needs of the patient. For instance, changing from an exoskeletal design, which is good for younger patients, to an endoskeletal design, may facilitate bicycle riding, as the potential for knee flexion is greater. Likewise, upgrading from a SACH to a SAFE foot improves hiking ability because of supplied subtalar action. Options that may appear trivial, such as "skin" color or toes versus no toes, may significantly increase the patient's satisfaction. Good prosthetic management optimizes children's functional level and enhances psychological and physical integration into their world.

It is hoped that amputation will be reserved for advanced disease in future.[33] Tumor resection with limb salvage procedures has become a safe and effective alternative to amputation.[34] The complexity of the limb salvage procedure is contingent upon the skeletal deficit following tumor resection.[31,33,34] Skeletal integrity is restored following femoral diaphyseal resection with a custom endoprosthesis or a vascularized fibular graft. A proximal femoral resection without joint involvement requires a segmental total hip replacement with a bipolar head. If a pelvic lesion is periacetabular, reconstruction is difficult and femoral fusion is indicated.

The proximal tibia and distal femur are the most prevalent sites for osteosarcoma.[35] The knee joint capsule, ligaments, and muscles are sacrificed, and a hinged total knee joint with a segmental prosthesis restores joint integrity and function. The quadriceps mechanism is preserved only if the patellar tendon can be reattached. A solid segmental arthrodesis, which produces a stable, pain-free weight-bearing extremity, is an alternative. Soft tissue coverage following knee joint resection may require primary or secondary transposition gastronemius flaps.[35] In the past younger children have been ineligible for limb salvage procedures owing to limb length discrepancy resulting from ongoing skeletal growth. However an adjustable internal prosthesis has been developed, which is periodically expanded surgically in order to maintain equal leg length.[36] An alternative for a femoral amputation in a growing child is a *rotationplasty*, in which the proximal tibia is rotated 180 degrees to replace the resected femur.[37] The ankle and foot are in a reversed position and now function as the knee joint. This allows further limb growth and converts an above-knee to a below-knee amputation.

The rehabilitative course following limb salvage is slow. Physical therapy management is specific to the type of orthopedic reconstruction involved. Although passive and active range-of-motion exercises are started early, weight bearing progression is often limited during the long engraftment period. In spite of the protracted rehabilitative course, limb salvage procedures are currently preferred to amputation.

EWING'S SARCOMA

Like osteosarcoma, Ewing's sarcoma is a highly malignant, anaplastic, predisseminated, primary bone tumor. It was first recognized as different from osteosarcoma by Ewing in 1921, when he observed vascular tumors arising in the bone marrow, and is devoid of any osteoid or chondroid matrix. Ewing reported that the incidence of this tumor in long and flat bone is almost equal and that extremity tumors involve the diaphysis. Although Ewing's sarcoma may arise anywhere in the skeleton, 60 percent of cases present in the extremities (more frequently lower than upper) including the femur (27 percent), tibia and fibula (17 percent), and humerus (16 percent). The remaining 40 percent involve flat bones, especially the pelvis (18 percent), vertebral body, and scapula.[38] The identity of the tumor cells that undergo transformation is unknown, and no etiologic clues have been discovered through either epidemiologic or animal studies.

Initial symptoms include local pain of short duration and possible swelling with or without a clinically appreciable mass. The tumor destroys the majority of the diaphysis and then spreads through the periosteum to form a large friable mass. As the tumor outgrows its blood supply, systemic symptoms occur, including fever, leukocytosis, anemia, increased sedimentation rate, and increased lactic dehydrogenase. Tumor is found to be disseminated in 20 percent or less of cases at diagnosis, but subclinical metastases are suspected in all cases. The tumor spreads to regional lymph nodes and travels hematogenously to lungs, bone marrow, and bone, especially the spine.

Owing to its vascular nature, Ewing's sarcoma is radiosensitive, tumoricidal doses being 50 to 60 Gy. Prior to the addition of systemic chemotherapy, radiation therapy was the sole treatment, and the 5-year survival rate was 10 percent. Chemotherapy trials with a combination of Adriamycin, actinomycin D, vincristin and Cytoxan, made as part of Intergroup Ewing's Sarcoma Study, have elevated 5 year survival rates to 50 to 80 percent.[39]

Traditionally, local tumor control has been achieved with radiation therapy delivering 30 to 40 Gy to the whole bone and a boost of 50 to 60 Gy to the tumor site. Some centers now advocate surgical resection of tumor so as to avoid complications of large-volume high-dose radiation, such as secondary malignancies, impaired bone growth, and pathologic fractures with delayed healing.[39]

Autologous bone marrow transplantation may be an option for patients with unfavorable disease (metastatic at diagnosis or a pelvic primary). The effect of bone marrow transplantation on long-term survival rates for poor prognosis patients has yet to be determined.[40]

Physical Therapy Management

The child with Ewing's sarcoma is followed by physical therapy from the time of initial diagnosis. Following excisional biopsy, a patient tends to limit movement of the affected joint because of pain. An appropriate exercise program is designed to preserve full joint mobility with minimal pain. Joint function must be further maintained throughout and beyond the course of radiation therapy, as joints within the radiation field are at risk for contracture secondary to radiation-induced fibrosis. As joint restriction may not be observed for several months, the exercise program must be carefully monitored on an ongoing basis so as to prevent joint dysfunction.

Children are prone to muscular underdevelopment, atrophy, and fibrosis following radiation therapy. The radiation therapy hinders replication of the highly nucleated sarcoplasm, whose rapid growth and increased volume are responsible for muscle bulk development. Although muscle may exhibit great deformity due to extensive radiation fibrosis, functional disturbance is often minimal in spite of severe atrophy. An exercise program for maximizing existing muscular strength is indicated, as progressive atrophy persists throughout the child's maturation.

As the entire involved bone is irradiated for local control of Ewing's sarcoma, pediatric skeletal growth alterations in the diaphysis, metaphysis, and epiphysis will occur. The degree of developmental disruption is directly proportional to the dose and volume of irradiation and inversely proportional to the patient's age. In the diaphysis, radiation alters periosteal activity, resulting in deficient bone modeling with decreased shaft width. The incidence of pathologic fracture is increased among patients with Ewing's sarcoma who have been treated by chemotherapy and irradiation, with the highest incidence in the femur followed by the humerus.[40] Fracture usually occurs months after cessation of treatment, and is not related to trauma. Early internal fixation with bone grafting is recommended, as radiation inhibits formation of endochondral and intramembranous bone, thereby jeopardizing callus formation and causing poor fracture union.

Abnormal absorption of calcified cartilage and bone causes metaphyseal alterations in the form of bowing, fraying, and abnormal tubulation. Hypoplastic changes are most evident in intramembranous bone with the greatest potential for development, including the orbit, mandible, and innominate bone. A hypoplastic acetabulum may be responsible for slipped capital femoral epiphyses and in the long term may lead to osteoarthritis, tendonitis, or bursitis.[41]

Radiation therapy causes epiphyseal damage by partially or completely sterilizing cartilaginous cells, which results in delayed or stunted longitudinal bone growth. Altered endochondral growth is compromised only when joints are irradiated. Growth may be arrested, remain delayed, or catch up to preirradiated growth rates. Limb length discrepancies are greatest during the two growth spurt periods of 2 to 6 years and adolescence. Skeletal growth limitations cannot be fully assessed until complete maturity is achieved.

Although disruption of bone growth induced by radiation therapy cannot be controlled, skeletal asymmetries are managed orthotically or surgically.[43] If the knee joint is included in the radiation field, leg length is greatly reduced, as 67 percent of lower extremity growth proceeds from the distal femur and proximal tibial growth plates. Leg length inequality must be corrected to avoid compensatory lumbar scoliosis, gait deficits, and long-term skeletal imbalances.

Leg shortening of less than 2 to 3 cm may be corrected with heel lifts. As leg length difference approaches 6 cm, decreasing ankle stability and increasing shoe weight place a limit on further orthotic correction, and surgical procedures should be considered. Shortening of the uninvolved leg may be accomplished by joint stapling or epiphysiodesis (creation of a bone bridge by realigning the growth plate). If limb discrepancy exceeds 6 cm, limb shortening is contraindicated because of compromise of muscle function and because of the resultant disproportionate appearance. Multiple limb lengthening procedures are indicated for discrepancies up to 15 cm, and greater discrepancies require amputation with prosthetic replacement.

RHABDOMYOSARCOMA

Rhabdomyosarcoma (RMS) is the most common and the most malignant of all pediatric soft tissue sarcomas. It accounts for 10 percent of all pediatric solid tumors and 6 percent of all pediatric malignancies, having a bimodal peak incidence at 2 to 6 years and 15 to 19 years. Genetic factors may contribute to RMS, as familial cases have been reported, and there is an increased incidence with breast cancer and with von Recklinghausen's disease. Although RMS has been induced in animals via viral and chemical agents, studies have been inconclusive in humans.

Because of its mesenchymal origin, RMS may occur in a variety of locations with a wide variety of clinical presentations. It has been classified according to three histologic categories—embryonal, alveolar, and pleomorphic. Embryonal RMS accounts for 50 to 65 percent of all cases, occurs in younger children, and is generally located in the head and neck, genitourinary tract, and abdomen. Botyroidal RMS, a variant of embryonal RMS, arises in hollow cavities (bladder and vagina). Alveolar RMS, constituting 20 percent of all cases, is the most differentiated, with striated muscle cells present, and may be associated with proliferation of muscle tissue in adolescence. It has a predilection for the 10- to 20-year age group and is found in peritoneum, perineum, and extremities (twice as frequently in the lower as in the upper). Pleomorphic RMS accounts for 1 percent of RMS cases, is rare in children, tends to occur in the 30 to 35 year age group, and is located in the trunk and extremities.

RMS presents deceptively as a small subcutaneous lump in the skin or in a more occult location. Symptoms are contingent upon tumor location and rate of growth. It follows the path of least resistance, extending locally, lymphatically, and hematogenously to lung and bone. Micrometastases are believed to be present in at least 90 percent of cases at diagnosis.

Medical management of RMS is difficult because of its complex histology and site presentation. The tumor is pseudoencapsulated, aggressively infiltrates local structures, and frequently has positive surgical margins. Radical surgery may be curtailed in sites such as the orbit and head and neck for functional and cosmetic reasons. Total en bloc resection is difficult and is performed in only one-third of cases. Disease is staged postoperatively based on tumor resectability as follows: stage I localized disease with complete resection (16 percent); stage II, localized disease with gross resection and residual microscopic disease (28 percent); stage III, gross unresectable disease (36 percent); and stage IV, distant metastatic disease (20 percent).

As total tumor extirpation is often not achieved, medical treatment includes a combination of chemotherapy and radiation therapy for both local and distinct tumor control.[43] Results of the Intergroup Rhabdomyosarcoma Study (IRS) clearly demonstrate that chemotherapy has significantly improved prognosis.[43] Ongoing IRS trials are designed to eliminate aspects of treatment that lack additional therapeutic value. The IRS has found that stage I disease responds equally to a combination of vincristin actinomycin D, and cyclophosphamide (VAC) and to VAC plus radiation therapy, with a 5-year survival rate in both groups of 85 percent. Postoperative radiation therapy is not required, does not improve survival rates, and may increase treatment complications. For stage II disease the 5-year survival rate is 72 percent with either vincristine-actinomycin D and radiation therapy or VAC treatment. Stage III and IV disease responds equally to VAC and radiation therapy or VAC with Adriamycin, survival rate for stage III being 57 percent and for stage IV 20 percent. Autologous bone marrow transplants are reserved for stage III and IV disease and recurrent disease. Interstitial radiation therapy using iridium 192 may be beneficial in hollow areas, as high-dose radiation may be delivered to small areas.[44]

The 5-year disease-free survival rate for all stages is 55 percent. By site the

5-year survival rates are orbit 84 percent, genitourinary and head and neck, 55 percent, extremities 47 percent, parameningeal sites 47 percent, and retroperitoneal sites 34 percent. Postrelapse survival rate is 32 percent at 1 year and 17 percent at 2 years.[43]

Physical Therapy Intervention

Physical deficits incurred in patients with RMS are similar to those seen in patients treated for Ewing's sarcoma. Physical therapy intervention involves postoperative mobilization, a long-term exercise program to minimize joint restriction and maximize muscle strength, and ongoing assessment and intervention to maintain skeletal alignment. Treatment toxicity is severe and often causes permanent deformity. The following case exemplifies progressive musculoskeletal sequelae requiring physical therapy intervention.

A 12-year-old girl had an alveolar RMS located in the right peroneal musculature. The 5-cm mass was grossly resected with wide margins (stage II). She was treated with chemotherapy (vincristine, Adriamycin, actinomycin D, and cyclophosphamide) and also received external-beam radiation therapy (60 Gy with the radiation field extending from the proximal knee to the malleoli with skin sparing).

The patient was initially referred to physical therapy owing to bilateral drop foot caused by vincristine neuropathy. Right ankle/toe weakness progressed with the onset of radiation fibrosis, culminating in an ankle contracture. As a leg length discrepancy evolved, the patient incurred ankle pain, balance and gait deficits, and a 20-degree thoracolumbar scoliosis.

During this period the patient received ongoing exercise and orthotic intervention to minimize leg and spine deficits. Owing to severe calf fibrosis and a leg length discrepancy of 6 cm, an Achilles tendon release and left knee stapling were required. The patient achieved good skeletal alignment with an ankle-foot orthosis and maintained ankle and knee stability with left and right sole modifications that equalized a 2-cm leg length discrepancy. The patient was instructed in a home exercise program to preserve ankle and paraspinal strength and flexibility. She was able to demonstrate a symmetrical gait and resumed participation in extracurricular sports.

CONCLUSION

Medical advances in the management of the pediatric patient with bone and soft tissue sarcoma have resulted in increased survival rates and in improved control of disease, thus permitting reduction in treatment and toxicity. As survival is becoming a reality for more children, the physical therapist must both address the immediate rehabilitative needs incurred during the cancer treatment period and anticipate future musculoskeletal sequelae. As dysfunction may evolve throughout the child's dynamic development period, it is imperative that ongoing physical therapy assessment and intervention be provided until developmental maturity is achieved.

REFERENCES

1. Rosenberg SA: Soft tissue sarcoma of the extremities. p. 1. In Sugarbaker PH, Nicholson TH (eds): Atlas of Extremity Sarcoma Surgery. JB Lippincott, Philadelphia, 1984
2. Rosenberg SA, Glatstein E: Perspectives on role of surgery and radiation therapy in the treatment of soft tissue sarcomas of the extremities. Semin Oncol 8:190, 1981
3. Rosenberg SA, Suit HD, Baker L, Rosen G: Sarcomas of the soft tissue and bone. p. 1036. In Devita VT, Hellman S, Rosenberg SA (eds): Principles and Practices of Oncology. JB Lippincott, Philadelphia, 1982
4. National Institutes of Health, Consensus Development Panel on Limb Sparing: Treatment of adult soft tissue sarcoma and osteosarcoma. JAMA 13:1791, 1985
5. Enneking WF: A system of staging musculoskeletal neoplasms. Clin Orthop 204:9, 1986
6. Eilber F, Guilano A, Huth J, et al: Limb salvage for high grade soft tissue sarcoma of the extremity; experience at UCLA. Cancer Treat Symp 3:49, 1985
7. Lampert MH, Gerber LH, Glatstein E, et al: Functional outcome in patients with soft tissue sarcoma of the extremity after wide local excision and radiation therapy. Arch Phys Med Rehabil 65:477, 1984
8. Shiu MH, Hajdu SI: Management of soft tissue sarcoma of the extremity. Semin Oncol 8:172, 1981
9. Brennan M, Shiu MH, Collen CS, et al: Extremity soft tissue sarcoma. Cancer Treat Symp 3:71, 1985
10. Shamberger RC, Sherins RT, Ziegler JJ, et al: Effects of postoperative chemotherapy and radiotherapy on ovarian function in women undergoing treatment for soft tissue sarcoma. JNCI 67:213, 1981
11. Shamburger RC, Sherins RT: Effects of postoperative chemotherapy and radiation in men undergoing treatment for soft tissue sarcoma. Cancer 47:2368, 1981
12. Suit HD, Wood WC, Proppe KH, Mankin HJ: Radiation therapy and conservative surgery for sarcomas of soft tissue. Prog Clin Cancer 8:311, 1982
13. Tepper JE, Suit HT: The role of radiation therapy in the treatment of soft tissue sarcoma. Cancer Invest 3:587, 1985
14. Enneking WF, McAuliffe JA: Adjunctive preoperative radiation therapy in treatment of soft tissue sarcoma. A preliminary report. Cancer Treat Symp 3:37, 1985
15. Waddington WW, Segraves KB, Simon MA: Psychological outcome of extremity sarcoma survivors undergoing amputation or limb salvage. Mayo J Clin Oncol 3:1393, 1985
16. Sugarbaker PH, Barofsky I, Rosenberg SA, Gianola F: Quality of life assessments of patients in extremity sarcoma clinical trials. Surgery 91:17, 1982
17. Lampert MH, Gerber LH, Sugarbaker PH: Rehabilitation of patients with extremity sarcoma. p. 33. In Sugarbaker PH, Nicholson TH (eds): Atlas of Extremity Sarcoma Surgery. JB Lippincott, Philadelphia, 1984
18. Sugarbaker PH: Alternative approaches to hemipelvectomy. p. 89. In Sugarbaker

PH, Nicholson TH (eds): Atlas of Extremity Sarcoma Surgery. JB Lippincott, Philadelphia, 1984

19. Sugarbaker PH, Lampert MH: Excision of quadriceps muscle group. Surgery 93:462, 1983

20. Malawer MM, Sugarbaker PH, Lampert MH, et al: The Tikhoff-Linberg procedure: Report of 10 patients and presentation of a modified technique for tumors of the proximal humerus. Surgery 97:518, 1985

21. Chang AE, Steinberg SM, Culnane M, et al: Functional and psychosocial effects of multimodality limb sparing therapy in patients with soft tissue sarcoma. J Clin Oncol 7:1217, 1989

22. Konrad JH, Ertl JE: Pediatric Oncology. Medical Examination Publishing, New York, 1978

23. Levine PA: Cancer in the Young. Masson Publishing, New York, 1982

24. Meyers PA: Malignant bone tumors in children: Hematol Oncol Clin North Am 1:655, 1987

25. Pritchard DJ: Factors that influence children that undergo amputation for bone of soft tissue sarcomas: The surgeon's viewpoint. NCI Monogr 56:133, 1981

26. Hockenberry MJ, Lane B: Limb salvage procedures in children with osteosarcoma. Cancer Nurs 11(1):2, 1988

27. Gill M, Murrells T, McCarthy M, Silcocks P: Chemotherapy for the primary treatment of osteosarcoma. Lancet 1:689, 1988

28. Gehbart MJ, Lane MD, Lane JM: Management of bone sarcomas at Memorial Sloan-Kettering Cancer Center. World J Surg 12, 299–306, 1988

29. Guilliland AE: Changing metastatic patterns of osteosarcoma. Cancer 54, 2160, 1984

30. Eilber FR, Eckhardt J, Morton DL: Advances in treatment of sarcomas of the extremity. Cancer 54:2695, 1984

31. Griffith ER: Rehabilitation of children with bone and soft tissue sarcomas: A physician's viewpoint. NCI Monogr 56:136, 1981

32. Nirenberg A: The adolescent with osteogenic sarcoma. Orthop Nurs 4(5):11, 1985

33. Makley JT, Krailo M, Ertel IJ, et al: The relationship of various aspects of surgical management in outcome in childhood cancer study group. J Pediatr Surg 23:146–151, 1988

34. Rao RN, Cammon JE, Pratt CB, et al: Limb salvage procedures for children with osteosarcoma: An alternative to amputation. J Pediatr Surg 15:901, 1983

35. Malawer MM, Price WM: Gastrocnemius transposition flap in conjunction with limb sparing surgery for primary bone sarcomas around the knee. Plast Reconstr Surg 73:741, 1984

36. Lewis MM: The use of an expandable and adjustable prosthesis in the treatment of childhood malignant bone tumors of the extremity. Cancer 57:499, 1986

37. Kotz R, Salzer M: Rotation-plasty for childhood osteosarcoma of the distal part of the femur. J Bone Joint Surg [AM]64:959, 1982

38. Meyers PA: Mailgnant bone tumors in children: Ewing's sarcoma. Hematol Oncol Clin North Am 1:667, 1987

39. Jurgens H, Exner O, Gadner H, et al: Multidisciplinary treatment of primary Ewing's sarcoma of bone. Cancer 61:21, 1988

40. Springfield PS: Fractures of long bones previously treated for Ewing's sarcoma. J Bone Joint Surg [AM]67A(3):477, 1985

41. Wolf EL: Slipped femoral capital epiphysis as a sequel to childhood irradiation for malignant tumors. Radiol, 125:781, 1977

42. Moseley CF: Unequal growth in children. In Ferguson AB Jr (ed): Orthopedic

Surgery in Infancy and Childhood. 5th Ed. Williams & Wilkins, Baltimore/London

43. Mauer HM, Beltongady M, Gehan EA, et al: The intergroup rhabdomyosarcoma study: A final report. Cancer 61:209, 1988
44. Ruymann FG: Rhabdomyhosarcoma in children and adolescents. Hematol Oncol Clin North Am 1:621, 1987
45. Sugarbaker PH, Nicholson TH: Atlas of Extremity Sarcoma Surgery. JB Lippincott, Philadelphia, 1984

7 | Psychosocial Issues in the Cancer Patient: Impact on Care

Julia H. Rowland

Since the late 1960s cancer has been transformed from what used to be an often fatal disease to a chronic, life-threatening illness, which has created an enormous challenge for patients, their families, and health care professionals alike. As the number of persons living with or cured of cancer has grown, so too has awareness of the special needs of this population with regard to physical, psychological, and social rehabilitation. Physical therapists are playing a growing role in the effort to help patients and their loved ones adjust to life after cancer. Their intense involvement in educating, training, and counseling patients places physical therapists in a unique position to provide a very special source of support and reassurance. In addition, because of the intensely personal nature of the work, the physical therapist serves as an extremely sensitive observer of a patient's level of distress and thus is in a position to identify patients who may need more specific interventions or additional support to achieve optimal recovery. For this reason it is important that the physical therapist have an understanding of the factors that contribute to psychological adaptation to cancer as well as of some specific areas that may need to be addressed.

This chapter briefly reviews the characteristics of the three major determinants to adaptation: the medical-related variables, the patient-related variables, and the sociocultural context. Specific psychological issues associated with rehabilitation from the cancers of specific anatomic sites discussed in this volume are then addressed. Finally, specific issues related to body-image and sexuality concerns, family interactions and staff stresses are discussed.

137

FACTORS IN ADAPTATION

Three sets of variables contribute to a patient's adaptation to cancer: medical-related issues,or those aspects of the disease and its treatment that affect outcome and potential quality of life; patient-specific issues, or what the patients brings to the illness in the way of resources or limitations; and sociocultural context, or how society views the illness and those treated (see Table 7-1).

Medical Variables

Clearly the stage at which cancer is diagnosed plays an important role in the patient's psychological response. Nevertheless, whether the prognosis is excellent or guarded, all patients must struggle with the uncertainty and will experience fluctuations, sometimes daily, in their ability to cope with the stresses of treatment and follow-up. Periods of maximal stress typically occur around the time of diagnosis; at the time of initial treatment; at any time of significant change in illness, treatment, or functional status; and at completion of treatment.[1] The latter point in particular can be overlooked. Rehabilitation team members need to be aware that patients may be more, not less, distressed at the anticipated end of therapy.[2] While team members may be happy for the progress made, the patient may see the end of therapy both as frightening and as representing the loss of a caring, supportive, and in a sense "protective" environment. The sense of vulnerability is heightened when treatment side effects cause the patient to feel worse than when therapy was initiated (e.g., following radiation for early-stage breast cancer). Plans should be made in advance to ease these transitions by discussing what will happen when treatment ends, reflecting that some people find this stressful, providing reassurance about continued staff availability, and scheduling an early follow-up visit to monitor ongoing progress.

Patients also report as stressful "anniversary" events such as the date at

Table 7-1. Primary Issues in Psychological Adjustment to Cancer

Determinants	Characteristics

Medical-related	Clinical facts
	  Stage and clinical course
	  Site of cancer
	  Nature of dysfunction/symptoms produced
	Treatment(s) required
	Rehabilitative options
	Psychological management by healthcare team

Patient-related	Intrapersonal
	  Age-specific developmental life tasks threatened/disrupted by cancer
	  Personality, prior coping skills, and illness/cancer experience
	Interpersonal
	  Nature/availability of social supports (family, friends, affiliated groups)

Sociocultural	Societal attitudes about cancer and the stigma and meaning attached

(From Holland and Rowland,[35] with permission.)

which they first found out they had cancer and the time around an annually scheduled follow-up. Acknowledging these as difficult periods for patients can help to diminish their fears and provide them with a sense of reassurance that they are not "going crazy."

The site of cancer and the nature of dysfunctions and symptoms produced affect psychological adaptation as well. Cancers that leave few permanent visible scars (e.g., leukemia and lymphoma) create fewer problems for social reentry than those whose treatment results in obvious physical impairment (e.g., sarcoma). However, even transient impairment such as hair loss can be devastating emotionally. Specific aspects of the psychological impact of treatment for cancers at specific sites addressed in this volume will be summarized in the sections that follow.

With the more aggressive approach to cancer control and cure it is likely that the patient will undergo a variety of treatments, the most common combination being surgery and chemotherapy. The consequence is that patients will often need rehabilitation for a variety of different medically related results or side effects. Because of the newness of some of these approaches there may be no assurance about the immediate or long-term sequelae. Therapists need to spend time discussing this issue with patients and allowing them to express their fears and concerns.

Whether the patient is informed about rehabilitative options and how this is accomplished has an important bearing on response to cancer.[3] Indeed, these issues may be the most critical in affecting psychological response to the medical variables. The patient who feels abandoned or who feels despairing of any quality of life after treatment will respond poorly to any attempt at subsequent rehabilitation. The growing emphasis on team care and early institution of rehabilitative efforts makes such an outcome increasingly rare.[4,5] Early exploration of a patient's beliefs about outcome and anticipated level of abilities is a critical task for the physical therapist.

Patient Variables

Three patient-related sets of variables affect psychological response to cancer (see Table 7-1). The first is the age or developmental stage at which the illness occurs. Each period in life has its own set of tasks to be achieved or mastered. Some of these are biologically determined (e.g., walking, puberty, menopause), some socially predicated (e.g., early schooling, voting, retirement), and others personally ascribed (e.g., marriage, becoming a senior executive, winning a specific award). When cancer strikes, achievement of these tasks and goals may be threatened or disrupted. Knowledge of what these are for each individual is important in planning rehabilitation not only for the immediate term but also with an eye to the future. For example, the young dancer who loses a leg to sarcoma will need support in her efforts to reset career goals and come to terms with lost aspirations. She may also need reassurance and counseling about feelings of disfigurement and concerns about her ability to attract and hold the interest of a sexual partner in the years to come. Knowing which tasks have been deferred or may not be achievable is important in the goal-setting process of rehabilitation.

The second patient-related variable of concern in assessing adaptation is the individual's prior coping experience. How the patient has responded to other life crises is often the single best indicator of how that patient will cope in the present. Hamburg and Adams have described the goals of effective coping behavior in serious illness as the ability to keep distress within manageable limits; maintain a sense of personal worth; restore close personal relationships; enhance prospects for recovery of physical functions; and increase the likelihood of working out a personally valued and socially acceptable situation after maximum physical recovery has been attained.[6] Researchers have found that those individuals who appear to cope best express an open acceptance of the cancer, exhibit a range of tackling behaviors, reflect active engagement with issues raised by diagnosis and treatment, and show flexibility in their use of coping strategies.[7,8] Brief exploration with a patient of coping responses and current reaction to illness is helpful in identifying the patient who is having trouble coping and needs referral for psychiatric or psychological consultation. As part of this evaluation, assessment of social support is also important, which brings us to the third factor in patient-related variables.[9]

Since the middle to late 1970s there has been a veritable explosion of research into the impact of social support on health. A positive relationship between social support and health or illness outcome is a consistent finding.[10] More specifically, considerable research exists to support the observation that the interpersonal environment of the person with cancer is of paramount importance in adapation.[11] Issues in the evaluation and management of family support will be discussed in greater detail later in the chapter.

Sociocultural Context

Since the late 1960s we in the United States have seen a reversal of the public's unwillingness to discuss illness in general and cancer in particular. The most dramatic evidence of the change in attitude is the greater willingness on the part of physicians to disclose a diagnosis of cancer.[12] In the last several years a number of public figures have disclosed treatment for cancer, from presidents and presidents' wives to well known actors, actresses, writers, and media figures. At a more subtle level, obituaries will now use the term "cancer" in place of the formerly often used phrase "lingering illness." The new openness has facilitated the adaptation of thousands of patients who can look to publicly acclaimed cancer survivors as role models for coping and can use the courage of these individuals to "go public." It has not eradicated, however, all the stigmas that still adhere to the disease, including illness-related job discrimination.

It is estimated that approximately 80 percent of treated cancer patients who were working previously will return to the workplace, but anywhere from 20 to 80 percent of these may experience work-related problems.[13] Feldman notes that negative attitudes on the part of the employer or co-workers and the survivor's self-attitudes may all conspire to make the reentered workplace a difficult setting after cancer treatment.[14] Employers may fear that the returned worker will be less productive, unable to match previous performance and more likely to be ill or absent. Employers are also concerned about the effect of the cancer patient on office morale and may fear that hiring or keeping on cancer survivors will increase company health and life insurance premiums. For their part, co-workers may erroneously fear that the disease is contagious or likely fatal and thus avoid contact with or restrict emotional support of the returned worker. Returning patients often have self-doubts about their ability to perform and worry about social rejection by co-workers and the possibility that the cancer might return. At the same time they may feel locked into a job by the dual threat that they would lose necessary insurance coverage if they quit or if their job were terminated and that with a history of cancer they might be unable to obtain a new position. As a result the workplace, often a vital source of self-esteem as well as financial security, becomes itself a source of stress.

In working with the patient each of these issues and concerns needs to be addressed. Preparation at reentry must deal with work stresses and with employers', co-workers', and family members' attitudes. An excellent forum for supportive counseling is a group in which other "veteran" patients with a similar or the same illness and treatments participate both as role models and as resources for problem solving. Expectation shaping and rehearsing can go a long way to decrease anxiety and bolster self-esteem by giving patients a chance to understand and anticipate problem areas while reinforcing a sense of confidence in their ability to handle difficult or distressing situations. Careful review of medical coverage plans as well as material available on employment rights of cancer survivors from the American Cancer Society should be encouraged. Referral to an employment or insurance counselor when necessary may be helpful.

In summary, a number of variables influence patient adaptation to cancer. Having an overview of these in mind when evaluating each new patient for rehabilitation is important. In their seminal work on the psychosocial adaptation of individuals to cancer, Weisman and Worden identified several factors that correlate with the presence (or absence) of distress following diagnosis.[7] Their index of vulnerability lists key indicators of risk that are helpful in evaluating and monitoring the recovering patient (Table 7-2).

SITE SPECIFIC PSYCHOLOGICAL RESPONSES

Head and Neck Tumors

The patient with a head and neck tumor faces a difficult rehabilitative course. Because of the inordinate emphasis our society places on both physical appearance and physical ability, the disabled or disfigured person, is often viewed as a deviant. Tumors of the head and neck region often result in the

Table 7-2. Indicators of Vulnerability to Poor Psychosocial Adjustment

Adjustment Areas	Indicators
Medical	More physical symptoms
	More advanced cancer at diagnosis
	Doctor perceived as less helpful
	Dubious about effect of treatment
	Short time perspective about survival
Psychological/ psychiatric	Premorbid psychiatric history; suicidal ideation
	High anxiety
	Low ego strength
	More suppression
	More concerns of all kinds
	Helpless/hopeless attitude
	Feels victimized or blames others for cancer illness
	Alcohol abuse
	Poorer coping skills
Social	Lower socioecomonic status
	More marital problems
	More frequent background problems
	Expects or receives little support from others
	Marginal or no church attendance

(Adapted from Weisman,[7] with permission.)

patient being labeled as both physically and visually impaired. The integrity of the face, especially the eyes, is vital to social interaction and emotional expression. Consequently, patients with tumors of the head are often reluctant to undergo surgery and are more likely than other surgical groups to be depressed postsurgery.[15] Reactions of others, fears of isolation and rejection, inability to hide disfigurement, and the loss of speech, sight, taste, smell or hearing, including at times subtle changes in a combination of these senses, can lead to crippling emotional reactions. Psychological impact appears to be directly related to the extent of disfigurement and sensory impairment. Postsurgical adjustment is further complicated by the high incidence of a premorbid history of chronic excessive alcohol or tobacco use.[16] Persons with a history of alcoholism tend to be dependent, have poor ability to change habits, and often manifest poor coping skills. Alcoholics, withdrawn suddenly from alcohol during hospitalization, may experience psychiatric symptoms (e.g., delirium tremens) postoperatively. The cognitive deficits and dementia associated with chronic alcohol consumption can compromise patients' ability to cooperate with or become involved in postoperative self-care. In addition, a number of chronic long-term sequelae of chronic alcoholism (e.g., family disruption, financial constraints) and the considerable risk of resumption of alcohol use put these patients at high risk for noncompliance and poor rehabilitative outcome. Individuals who used alcohol and/or tobacco to control stress are likely to experience heightened anxiety and distress with discontinuation and abstinence.

Loss of ability together with loss of pleasure from such intrinsic activities as eating and speaking can be devastating. Many patients who receive radiation to the head also report taste changes, which in some cases do not reverse over time and which render unpalatable many previously enjoyed foods. Use of patient volunteers or "veteran" patients for counseling may provide a uniquely successful adjunct to supportive care among patients treated for head and neck malignancies. Knowing that there are others who have been through the same experience and can serve as sympathetic supporters and role models is reassuring. These individuals are often a source of information and helpful hints on handling not only embarrassing social situations but also more mundane difficulties such as those arising from loss of vital functions (e.g., ability to speak on the phone for the laryngectomy or partial glossectomy patient). Self-help groups such as the laryngectomee associations supported by the American Cancer Society or the Lost Chords, another national organization, have grown up to meet the special needs of this treatment group and should be considered in treatment plans. A newer organization called Let's Face It, located in Concord, Massachusetts, provides a network for people with facial disfigurement from any cause, not necessarily cancer. They see their goal as linking people with facial disfigurement, their families and friends, and professionals with resources for recovery. Referral for further psychiatric assessment or psychological support as necessary is important in efforts to ensure full rehabilitation. This intervention should always be considered where there is a premorbid history of alcohol abuse or psychiatric problems. In addition, Breitbart and Holland emphasize that if the patient's background places a premium on physical appearance (e.g., model, company representative) or communication skills (e.g., salesperson, teacher, public speaker), special counseling is warranted.[15]

A series of studies looking at predictors and correlates of adaptation to head and neck cancer provide additional information helpful in anticipating rehabilitation needs. Dropkin and colleagues found that delay in assuming self-care responsibilities beyond postoperative day 5 or 6 was predictive of poor coping and poor rehabilitative outcome.[17] They also noted that those individuals with a high need for approval proceed more slowly. A report by Natvig evaluating laryngectomees found that good premorbid adjustment was highly predictive of ability to adapt to loss of laryngeal speech and to mastery of esophageal speech.[18] High motivation of both patient and family and realistic expectations from the speech rehabilitation program have also been shown to be predictive of good vocational and social adjustment.[19]

Despite the multiple handicaps to recovery experienced by head and neck patients, they have as a group been shown to adapt remarkably well. In a survey by West, 95 percent of 152 disfigured patients reported good social, vocational, and interpersonal adjustment.[20] Recognition that they were cured was cited as a significant determinant in ability to accept the losses consequent to treatment.

Lung Cancer

Several aspects of the etiology and treatment of lung cancer are of particular concern regarding the psychological response of patient and family to a diagnosis of this disease. First is the recognition that the majority of lung cancers

(85 percent in men, 75 percent in women) are related to cigarette smoking. Viewed from an epidemiologic perspective, this means that lung cancer is the single most preventable tumor. Despite this, smoking cessation campaigns and campaigns to prevent adolescents from taking up the habit have been difficult.[21] Individuals who present with a smoking history frequently feel considerable guilt about having caused their illness themselves; this guilt is often compounded by a sense of blame that is placed on the victim, consciously or not, by the health professional, family, and society. Persons who develop lung cancer as a result of industrial exposure to carcinogens such as asbestos may feel anger. The minority of patients who develop the disease despite having no known risk factors may resent the perceived assumption by others that they smoked or somehow caused their illness.

Added to the common burden of self-blame is awareness that the long-term prognosis for this disease is generally poor. Only 13 percent of all lung cancer patients are alive 5 or more years after diagnosis, and survival rates have increased only slightly since the late 1970s.[22] The reason for these poor survival figures is that diagnosis is difficult and most patients present with advanced disease.

As a consequence of these two aspects, patients with lung cancer may be at increased risk for depression and hopelessness. A study by Hughes in England of patients presenting with suspicious symptoms revealed that 16 percent exhibited major depressive symptoms prior to hearing the diagnosis, which suggests that some patients are likely aware of the seriousness of their situation even before a cancer diagnosis is made.[23] It is important for physical therapists to have an understanding of how patients perceive their illness and to monitor their own feelings about causation in working with patients. Working with those whose addiction to cigarettes is strong and who continue to smoke can be particularly stressful. If patients perceive the therapist as blaming or pessimistic, their willingness to engage in rehabilitative efforts will be minimal.

Two additional medical features of this disease with psychological ramifications that complicate rehabilitation are the presence of metastatic disease and the potential for development of paraneoplastic syndromes.[21] Brain metastases occur in approximately 30 to 40 percent of patients with lung cancer.[24] These may result in changes in personality and behavior as well as in cognition as reflected in slowed thinking and memory impairment. Treatment of brain metastases, whether primary or prophylactic, in particular when it involves cranial irradiation, may also result in changes in mentation and behavior.[25] Patients with lung cancer are also vulnerable to developing paraneoplastic syndromes, which by indirect effect on other systems can affect neuropsychologic functioning. Of particular importance are the endocrine and neurologic-myopathic syndromes, which can produce psychiatric symptoms and dementia, respectively.

Problems in understanding or remembering instructions need to be anticipated in patients who have brain disease or who develop paraneoplastic syndromes. In such cases it is helpful to supplement sessions with lists or written instructions concerning programmed exercises and to enlist a family member's help in encouraging and carrying out homework assignments. Physical therapists, because of their daily work with patients, may be among the first to detect subtle changes that suggest progression of disease or development of a treatment side effect. Therapists working with lung cancer patients need to be alert to the potential for development of behavioral or mental changes and to report any observed alterations to the attending physician for further workup. Therapists should also be aware that anxiety can increase dyspnea in these patients. When this occurs, panic may set in and further exacerbate the situation. Attention to symptoms of anxiety and teaching techniques that enable lung cancer patients to relax before starting exercises are important in ensuring their ability to carry out proposed exercises or to continue efforts.

Problems of weight loss, pain, weakness, shortness of breath, and cough, which often persist after treatment, can strain efforts to maintain psychological equilibrium. Nevertheless, studies have shown that many patients are able to do well despite the seriousness of their disease. Driever and McCorkle found that although lung cancer patients exhibited poorer physical status and greater severity of symptoms, they were able to maintain as positive an attitude as a comparison group of patients who had experienced myocardial infarction.[26] In an earlier study among advanced lung cancer patients cared for at home, a similar pattern of response was found.[27] In spite of advancing symptoms and diminishing physical status, this group also showed a largely optimistic attitude. Of particular interest is the more recent research by Cella and colleagues,[28] in which patients being treated for small cell lung cancer were assessed by the Profile of Mood States, a self-report of mood, prior to commencing chemotherapy. It was found that when performance status was good, total mood disturbance or distress was low regardless of extent of disease. The researchers interpreted these results as suggesting that patients' knowledge of disease, even when extensive, is less distressing in the absence of disabling symptoms. They emphasized, however, that the common concurrence of physical symptoms and awareness of the severity of disease is predictive of greater distress in lung cancer patients.

While reports of psychological studies among lung cancer patients are still few, a small literature of hopeful personal accounts available to patients and families struggling with this disease is beginning to accumulate. In particular are the articles by Alice Trillin, a long-term survivor of lung cancer and wife of the well known writer Calvin Trillin, and that of R.M. Mack, a surgeon who writes intelligently and sensitively about his experience with initial complete remission and subsequent recurrence.[29,30]

Breast Cancer

No other anatomic site has received more attention with respect to the psychological impact of cancer than the breast cancer. Indeed, breast cancer is often used as a paradigm for understanding psychological adaptation to cancer; thus much of what has been found in breast cancer is often applied to our understanding of what it is like to be a cancer patient or family member or health professional supporting these patients.

Much has changed since the late 1960s in the understanding and treatment

of breast cancer. Previously, little was discussed with the patient preoperatively, mastectomy was almost uniformly the treatment of choice, and women
were frequently sent home with assurances that the surgeon had "got it all."
Today women have a choice of options with regard to primary treatment, are
often given explicit information about the nature and extent of their disease
(including the fact that there are no guaranteed cures and follow-up is for life),
and are encouraged to be active participants in their full care and recovery.
While taboos still exist, the disclosure of their experience with breast cancer by
public figures such as Betty Ford, Nancy Reagan, and Gloria Steinem has
increased public awareness of and advocacy on behalf of survivors of this
disease. In addition, many more supports are available to women coping with
breast cancer, from a growing list of local and community support groups to
national resources such as the American Cancer Society's Reach to Recovery
program and the National Alliance of Breast Cancer Organizations (NABCO),
an information clearinghouse based in New York City.

Despite wide variability in methodology, studies of adapation to mastectomy reveal a remarkable consistency in women's concerns: confrontation with
a potentially fatal disease; impact of the loss of breast on body image and
appearance; diminished sense of femininity; decrease in sexual attractiveness
and function; fear of recurrence; and shame and guilt. Mourning for the loss of a
cherished body part and the threat to life are universal, but the extent to which
they are experienced is highly variable. Earlier studies suggested that anywhere
from 10 to 56 percent of women suffered some degree of impairment of social or
emotional function postmastectomy.[31] A more recent study using a large prospective sample and controlling for premorbid psychiatric history did not find
serious psychiatric sequelae at 1 year post-treatment.[32] Although breast cancer
patients exhibited more distress related to social and interpersonal relationships, quality of life was equal to that of unaffected peers. In this study it was
observed that women with stage II disease who received adjuvant chemotherapy had higher levels of distress throughout the 12-month study. Physical therapists need to be aware of the greater support needs in this group of patients.
Clinical experience, as well as the picture presented in the work of Bloom and
co-workers,[32] suggests that breast cancer patients frequently experience a cur-
vilinear pattern in their psychological response to illness. After a peak distress
period around the time of diagnosis, some stabilization of emotions is reached
during and immediately after treatment. It is not uncommon, however, to note
an increase in symptoms of distress 3 to 6 months postsurgery. This coincides
with recovery from surgery and radiation and the time of resumption of full
activities. Recognition by staff and reassurance of the patient and family when
such reactions occur are helpful in limiting more serious distress.

The availability of breast-conserving approaches to treatment and of reconstructive surgery to address cosmetic concerns have done much to reduce the
psychic trauma associated with loss of the breast. Although some women find
the decision-making process an extremely difficult one, research carried out
several months after treatment was completed suggested that most women are
happy with the choice they made.[33] Other studies have indicated, nevertheless,

that differing characteristics of individual patients may lead them to select different options in those cases in which choices are offered. Women choosing limited resection and radiation (versus mastectomy) appear to be more concerned about potential insult to their body image, more dependent on their breasts for self-esteem, and more likely to believe that they would have difficulty adjusting to loss of the breast. Patients selecting mastectomy more often perceive the cancer-containing breast as foreign and want to have it removed; they also express more fears about the potentially harmful effects of radiation.[34] One consequence of these differences between groups is that women who opt for breast conservation and whose cosmetic result following surgery and radiotherapy is less than desired may be at significant risk for anger and depression.

A small subgroup (less than 10 percent) of women undergoing mastectomy will choose to pursue the option of breast reconstruction. In the past these women have appeared very similar to their peers who did not choose reconstruction with respect to levels of self-esteem, feelings of attractiveness, sexual functioning, or self-reported psychological symptoms.[35] They did report greater discomfort with their external prosthesis and attached greater importance to their breasts. The reasons most frequently cited for seeking surgery were to be rid of the prosthesis, to "feel whole again," and to reestablish symmetry and thus diminish self-consciousness about appearance. These studies, however, were conducted at a time when breast conservation was not as widely available as today. It is likely that many women selecting reconstruction in the past would have selected breast conservation had it been available. It is nevertheless important to realize that even if the patient does not choose to pursue this as an option, knowing that she might be a candidate for such surgery in the future restores a sense of control over her situation and can be extremely helpful to her adjustment. This may be of particular value if the woman desires breast conservation but is, for medical reasons, a poor candidate.

Although women undergoing breast-sparing techniques appear in the early post-treatment period (3 to 6 months) to have fewer problems with body image and sexual comfort and satisfaction, studies of the overall psychological adjustment of breast cancer patients have found few differences between treatment groups (mastectomy, mastectomy plus reconstruction, and limited resection and radiation.)[36] Indeed, some researchers feel that the emotional benefit associated with breast-conserving surgery relative to more radical surgery has been less than expected.[37] It has been noted by clinicians that some women undergoing limited resection may, because of the less radical extent of their surgery, feel that they had a "milder" case of cancer and exhibit greater denial of the seriousness of their illness. For these women it may not be until initiation of radiation, with its attendant daily visits and cumulative feelings of fatigue, that they feel the full emotional impact of the illness and experience a renewed sense of fear and concern about the nature of their disease and treatment. Therapists should be alert to these delayed reactions. It has also been observed—and voiced as a concern by patients themselves—that because they have not lost their breasts, staff and family believe that they need less support. Often the contrary is true given the extended length of treatment imposed by radiation. From a rehabilitative point of view, it is the axillary dissection, surgery common to both mastectomy and resection patients, that poses the most difficulties in postsurgical recovery.

An extremely effective model of rehabilitation for breast cancer patients has been used for many years at Memorial Sloan-Kettering Cancer Center.[38] All patients undergoing breast cancer surgery are asked to participate in weekday meetings during their postsurgical stay. The meetings, coordinated jointly by nursing and social work staff, include a review of the psychological impact of breast cancer, its physical effects, and exercises. The exercise program is demonstrated and supervised by a physical therapist. In addition, women meet a trained patient volunteer who talks about prostheses and serves as a role model for adaptation. This multimodal approach, with repeat sessions, is extremely helpful in addressing the woman's comprehensive needs. The group format fosters mutual support, reinforces learning, and helps to ensure that important questions are asked and clearly answered.

Encouragement of spouses and partners in special weekly group meetings is an integral part of the rehabilitative program at Memorial Sloan-Kettering as well. Wellisch and colleagues have documented the importance of the spouse's involvement in decision making and inpatient recovery to later marital adjustment.[39] Early viewing of the scar is helpful in promoting adjustment. As with the patient who has undergone head and neck surgery, the woman who refuses to look at her surgical site, is reluctant to participate in self-care, or reports several months after surgery that she still wears a brassiere or cover-up garment at all times, even in bed, may warrant referral to the mental health member of the team. For women who have undergone mastectomy, finding a comfortable, well-fitting prosthesis is vital to reestablishing a sense of self-esteem and femininity. Making available to patients a list of shops that cater to the special needs of mastectomy patients is extremely useful.

Leukemia/Lymphoma

The epidemiologic characteristics of the different diseases that constitute the adult leukemias and lymphomas and specifically the age at diagnosis present different psychological management issues. While non-Hodgkin's lymphoma, whose peak incidence is between ages 40 and 70, affects a broad spectrum of adults, leukemia and Hodgkin's lymphoma patients represent the two extremes of the adult age range. The fact that almost 90 percent of adults diagnosed with leukemia are over age 60 has several psychological ramifications for patient and health care provider alike. As medical advances increase life span and health among older adults, it is increasingly difficult to generalize about this segment of the population. Nevertheless, specific changes in physical and social circumstances are expected to occur in later decades, although there is great variability in the impact produced by these in different individuals. As a consequence of aging, rehabilitative efforts may take longer, produce more fatigue, and result in lower achieved levels of performance than might be expected for younger patients with comparable dysfunction at presentation. In addition, the older adult is more vulnerable to chronic medical conditions such as heart disorders or renal failure that further compromise recuperative efforts. These natural limitations can be extremely frustrating to older patients for whom regaining previous levels of independence and function may seem painfully slow or unattainable; the therapist may at times believe that the patient has "given up."

At the same time that they are experiencing and adapting to physical losses, older adults may also be adjusting to social losses such as: widowhood, retirement, restricted finances, loss of or moving away from a family home, and death of friends and relatives. Managing the stress of cancer in the context of multiple losses can lead to depression; patients over 70 may be particularly vulnerable.[40] Absence of friends and family also deprive them of a vital support system necessary for full recuperation. Finally, because of their physical vulnerability, older patients are more likely to experience mental compromise owing to the direct or indirect effects of the cancer and its treatment. In their review of 546 patients referred for psychiatric consultation at Memorial Sloan-Kettering, Holland and Massie found that patients 60 and older were twice as likely to receive a diagnosis of organic mental disorder as younger patients.[40]

Although they are at increased risk for specific psychological difficulties, older adults can draw on special strengths. Studies have shown that older patients may adapt better to chronic or life-threatening illness than younger patients.[41,42] Cassileth and colleagues surmise that differences in coping may reflect the fact that older patients have developed more effective stress management skills; illness in the older patient may also result in increased attention and involvement with others, offsetting the negative impact on physical function.[41] Ganz et al. postulate that greater experience with illness and prior hospitalizations enables older patients to communicate better with the medical team and to report less psychological and social distress than younger patients.[43] The greater ability of older adults to adapt to illness may also reflect anticipation of illness and death associated with advancing age. While life-threatening illness is never welcome, it is expected in old age but not in the young.

In working with the older patient, the physical therapist needs to be aware of these strengths and vulnerabilities. Establishing clear, realistic goals of rehabilitation based on prior levels of function with planned rates of progression that encourage patients but do not leave them helpless is important. Provision of guidelines in straightforward terms, with written and repeated presentations, is helpful in minimizing any confusion arising from impaired vision or hearing. Maisiak and colleagues found that older patients were more likely than younger to miss appointments because of lack of faith in the treatments and, importantly, dislike of the confusing clinic atmosphere.[42] Physical therapists should be alert to mental changes in their older patients as these may be a first sign of organ failure or secondary complications of disease or treatment. In addition, assessment of the adequacy of a patient's social support system and bolstering this as needed should be part of follow-up. It should be added that many health professionals find that the older patient with advanced cancer is easier to work with than the younger.

In contrast to adult leukemia, Hodgkin's disease is a young adult cancer. As such it brings with it age-related issues, in particular the unexpected and unwanted confrontation with death. Progress in curing Hodgkin's disease represents one of the great success stories in oncology since the late 1960s. Although it was once a uniformly fatal disorder, the 5-year survival rate for patients diagnosed today at ages under 35 is 80 percent. Cure, however, is effected with highly toxic, lengthy, and demanding chemotherapeutic regimens. The young adult, struggling to complete advanced educational degrees and to achieve career, interpersonal, and family goals is severely stressed by a cancer diagnosis. Becoming dependent upon a medical system at a time when establishment of independence is expected sets young patients apart from their peers, producing feelings of diminished self-esteem and competency. Placement of Broviac or Hickman lines to ease care imposes on these patients a high technical level of self-care and compliance. Working with a team whose members are often of a similar age can produce anger and resentment in patients and anxiety and defensiveness in team members, which can interfere with optimal care. A premium is often placed on working out a treatment schedule that minimizes family and work disruption, a goal that may conflict with busy clinic and staff demands.

Pressure to resume usual responsibilities in this young group, whether internally or externally imposed, can lead to overly ambitious goal-setting, making patients susceptible to failure and disappointment when they find themselves unable to achieve desired levels of activity. In extreme cases this can result in actual physical compromise, as with patients who press forward too quickly, thus taxing rather than strengthening muscles, tissue, and stamina. The physical therapist needs to be sensitive to all these issues in organizing and delivering care to the young adult. Acknowledging frustration while reviewing periodically and supporting appropriate speed of recovery reduces the likelihood of disappointment and setbacks.

Leukemia and lymphoma share several aspects in that certain psychological reactions that may occur when therapy ends are common to both groups of patients. First, because these illnesses often present initially with minor symptoms, patients may exhibit high anxiety when changes in appearance or function are experienced. This is particularly true for any symptom that mimics those experienced at time of cancer diagnosis (e.g., fever, swollen glands, fatigue). Reassurance by the treating physician is important along with support from the team for establishing a new and appropriate level of "body monitoring." Second, a large number of patients experience profound fatigue and diminished stamina long after treatment has ended.[44] Explaining that this may be a latent side effect and encouraging patience with self should be part of the rehabilitative process. Third, because of the length and intensity of the treatment they receive, these patients, more than other groups of adult cancer survivors, are at risk for difficulties in discarding the patient role and returning to normal. The duration of the disruption, the habit of restructuring activities of daily living around illness, and the life and death dependence on the medical team during care make subsequent separation very difficult. Plans to ease this transition should be in place long before treatment stops.

Sarcoma

Although the need for inclusion of a physical therapist as a member of the treatment team may be variable in the care of some cancer patients, physical therapists are integral to the treatment and recovery of patients with osteogenic sarcoma. As with head and neck cancer patients, in whom dramatic changes in appearance and ability are often an anticipated outcome of treatment, involvement of the physical therapist early in the planning of care is critical. Preparing the patient and family for what to expect following surgery and outlining a rehabilitative program promotes hope and encourages active involvement. Visits during the planning stage also afford the therapist an opportunity to observe the patient's appearance and assess premorbid level of functioning. A visit prior to surgery by a patient who has had similar surgery and is doing well can also be helpful.

Regardless of the type of tumor or age of the patient, loss of a limb or body part is accompanied by an expected and necessary mourning period. The intensity of the grief expressed is very variable. However, if it continues unabated beyond 6 months or if maladaptive coping patterns (e.g., withdrawal, apathy, extreme denial, hyperactivity) emerge, referral for further psychiatric evaluation is essential.

With osteogenic sarcoma as with Hodgkin's disease, the age of presentation, with a peak incidence between 10 and 25 years, requires an understanding of developmental issues. While younger children may not fully comprehend the life-threatening nature of their illness, the adolescent not only understands the threat to life posed by cancer but also appreciates the abstract uncertainty of long-term survival. The normal tasks of adolescence—puberty, achieving independence, identity formation, peer conformity/acceptance, early exploration of intimate interpersonal relationships—are in direct conflict with the demands imposed by chronic illness. As a consequence, illness during this developmental period can lead at times to a struggle between extremes—a regressive pull to be nurtured and taken care of, and a tendency to denial, acting out, and noncompliance. In research by Smith and colleagues, up to 59 percent of adolescent cancer patients assessed were found to be noncompliant with some aspect of their therapies.[45] Although this study focused on medication-related compliance, it is likely that prescribed physical activities are equally vulnerable to omission in this group.

Monitoring for maladaptive responses is important. However, evaluations need to take into account the expected normal independent strivings of this population. Indeed, perhaps more than in other age groups monitoring for the "too good" (quiet, compliant, uncomplaining) adolescent patient is important. At an age where some opposition is expected, deviation in the opposite extreme may serve as a red flag for depression. Acknowledging adolescents' fears and concerns, involving them in the planning of treatment and rehabilitation, empathic limit setting, and discussion of techniques to manage anxiety-producing situations (e.g., peer group interactions) are important in promoting adaptive coping. Use of peer patient groups is also helpful, with the option of referral for short-term psychotherapy available as needed. A unique rehabilitative program has been developed at the Hospital for Special Surgery in New York City. Referred to as ASPIRE (Adolescent Sarcoma Patients' Intense Rehabilitation with Exercise), the program, which combines special prosthetic development, intensive rehabilitation, fitness training, and counseling, promotes physical as well as emotional and social recovery of amputees. Program participants ranked among some of the award winners in the eighth Paralympic Games held in Seoul after the Summer Olympics in 1988.

Management of pain in the cancer patient is always a concern. It is further complicated in the care of the adolescent and young adult patient owing to physician biases in pain assessment,[46] developmentally related distortion in reporting pain,[47] and denial or minimization of new pain whether through concern about its potential implications (fear of recurrence, graft rejection) or because of a need to feel in control of the situation.[48] Knowledge of these differences in perception and reporting of pain is important to the physical therapist, who may use pain level to evaluate efficacy of planned interventions.

Studies of the long-term adjustment of osteogenic sarcoma patients to school, work, and social, sexual and family life indicates they are successful in achieving independence despite acknowledged difficulties in mobility.[49,50] Nor does it appear that psychiatric morbidity is increased among amputees as contrasted to healthy peer groups.[51] When prolonged or severe psychological disruption occurs, referral for further assessment is indicated. Introduction of limb-sparing approaches to treatment since the late 1960s has sought to address some of the latent psychological morbidity associated with amputation. Despite the greater complexity of the surgery, risk of infection, and cosmetic and rehabilitative demands, limb salvage is being used increasingly in some centers. The assumption is that by avoiding loss of the body part, body integrity is preserved and psychological adaptation enhanced. There is some debate, however, as to whether this is the case. Kagan found that emotional adjustment may be more difficult for limb salvage patients because of the longer hospitalizations and uncertain outcome.[48] Two additional studies have failed to demonstrate differences in quality of life and physical and psychological measures between limb salvage and limb amputation patients.[49,51] It must be anticipated that postoperative distress will be higher for patients who anticipate limb salvage but for whom amputation is deemed necessary at the time of surgery. As with any new procedure, long-term follow-up of patients will be necessary to determine the relative advantages of salvage versus amputation and whether the individual characteristics of some patients suggest that they might be better served by undergoing one or the other treatment.

GENERAL CONSIDERATIONS
Sexual Concerns

Few rehabilitation texts available today fail to acknowledge that all persons with cancer need sexual information, counseling, and support from the treatment team. The emotional distress, pain, fatigue, and insult to the patient's body image and self-esteem caused by the diagnosis and treatment of cancer may severely damage sexual functioning, even among individuals who had a strong and satisfying sexual relationship prior to illness. When illness occurs in the context of preexisting problems, the outcome may be devastating. Despite heightened sensitivity to sexual issues, in practice provision of effective sexual interventions is highly variable, often because of staff avoidance.

Auchincloss has found that staff resistance or reluctance to address patients' sexual concerns cluster around four broad themes.[52] First, many professionals whose focus is on treatment and management of illness feel the sexual consequences of treatment are not their concern. Auchincloss argues strongly that, as with any other side effect of treatment, the responsibility for monitoring sexual sequelae rests with the oncology team. Second, many staff members are reluctant to raise the topic of sex because they feel that little information is available to remedy problems. This attitude is being slowly replaced as the field of sex therapy has grown. Education about effective therapies for problems such as impotence, painful intercourse, and lack of desire is acknowledged and currently available. Third, belief that the patient is principally (or solely) concerned with his cancer prevents other staff from raising sexual issues. Work by Vincent and colleagues challenges the accuracy of this perception. In their study, 80 percent of patients interviewed desired more information about sexual issues, although 75 percent expressed reluctance to broach the subject themselves.[53] Finally, some staff personnel may simply feel too embarrassed to discuss sex. Auchincloss stresses that with time, education, patience, and practice, most health professionals can come to believe that they have something to offer patients who are anxious, distressed over new problems, and unsure of how to go about asking for help. She emphasizes that caregivers should be reassured that patients often feel an enormous sense of relief to have a problem acknowledged, to know that it is not uncommon, and that help is available through suitable referral.[52]

In short, it is the staff's obligation to raise the issue of potential or actual impact of illness and treatment on this area of function and to discuss sexual rehabilitation options with every patient from the adolescent to the elderly. Patients who are young or single and those whose treatment directly affects sexual response are at particular risk for problems in sexual function and deserve special attention.

Sexual rehabilitation starts ideally before treatment with a good social and sexual history. With regard to patients for whom impairment of sexual function might be anticipated (e.g., infertility in leukemia patients), discussion of these effects is essential. Raising the topic of sexual function early by letting the patient know it is an appropriate focus of concern and that the health care provider is willing to discuss it opens the door for future dialogue in this area and helps to ensure that problems with sexual function will be addressed. Auchincloss cautions, however, against initiating sexual discussions during periods of acute stress (e.g., treatment setbacks, recurrences, family or work crises) and places a high premium on finding a private space for conducting such interviews.[52]

Some teams may wish to designate one staff member to initiate conversations or to follow up on those introduced by the primary physician. It is important to establish this role, as it is as undesirable to have everyone asking about sexual function as to have no one address this area. Above all, it is necessary for the team members to know about efforts in this area and to coordinate their input with that of others. When specific questions arise, physical therapists need to know what the patient has been told and by whom so that they can serve to focus questions for patients, direct their inquiries to the appropriate staff member, clarify or reinforce information provided, and serve as advocates for the patients.

It is beyond the scope of this chapter to go into the particular types of problems that may occur or their treatment. There are, nevertheless, a number of excellent resources in the growing field of sexual rehabilitation of cancer patients.[54,55] Among these are two excellent manuals for patient use entitled *Sexuality and the Woman who has Cancer and Her Partner,* and *Sexuality and the Male who has Cancer and His Partner;* both are available through the American Cancer Society. In addition, there are now a small number of programs around the country that train sex counselors and therapists, and names of qualified sex therapists are available for referral or workshop purposes from the American Association of Sex Educators, Counselors and Therapists, based in Washington, D.C.

Physical therapists, by the very nature of their work, deal daily with issues of body image and sexuality. Intense hands-on contact with their patients and daily assessments of physical function and performance afford them a natural opportunity to monitor problems in sexual function and to support sexual rehabilitative efforts. By encouraging patients to be comfortable with their bodies and to ask questions about abilities and changes and by modeling and reflecting back to their patients self-approval, body esteem, and a sense of personal attractiveness and social acceptability, physical therapists can contribute significantly to the healing process.

Family Issues

It is probably a truism to state that the physical therapist's greatest ally in rehabilitative efforts is the family. Less frequently acknowledged—but no less true—is the fact that the family can also be a major source of conflict in efforts to provide optimal patient care. As noted earlier in this chapter, the impact of social support on health and illness has become an area of keen interest. Although specific aspects of support have proved more helpful than others, the overall finding in studies involving cancer patients is that degree of social support is positively associated with both better adjustment and longer survival.[56]

When people are ill, they tend to feel less in control, less powerful, and more inferior, especially when they must rely on others. At the same time serious illness of any kind increases the ill person's need for closeness to others to counteract feelings of insecurity and vulnerability. The need for love and support often heightens in patients over time, both as a reaction to the effects of disease and treatment and the fear that they will no longer be loved or cared for. Fears of abandonment and rejection, experienced by other critically ill patients, are often keenly felt by the cancer patient.

Active involvement of the family clearly serves a range of patient needs— from the most basic, namely, provision of emotional support (the "psychic fuel" that keeps a patient going), to the practical (e.g., transportation to therapy sessions and financial resources to support these services), to the more abstract (e.g., providing meaningful roles and hence functional goals toward which the patient can strive). For their part, physical therapists may count on the family member to be an advocate, a home trainer, and a one-person cheering section on the behalf of the patient—in short, to be a partner in accomplishing the goals set in rehabilitation. The vital nature and complexity of the relationship of spouse and family to patient well-being is no more obvious than when this system goes awry.

When such situations occur, it is critical to remember that support is a two-way street; the source of the problem may arise in the provider of support (family member) as well as in the recipient (patient) and commonly involves both (see Table 7-3). The impact of cancer can be as devastating to a family member as to the patient himself. Spouses may feel angry, ashamed, and vulnerable to illness themselves. Clinicians working with families of cancer patients suggest that they may at times need to be viewed as second-order patients.[57] Seeing that spouses have a support network and chance to air conflicting emotions can be critical to ensuring that they will be available to patients when needed. Toward this end staff persons need to acknowledge the difficult task faced by spouses, to provide opportunities for them to talk about feelings both with patients and alone with staff people, and to ensure that backup supports are available and provision is made to give the spouse time off. While encouraging

Table 7-3. Problem Sources in Obtaining and Maintaining Adequate Social Support in Illness

Problem Source	Types of Issues
Provider	Availability
	Emotional
	Physical
	Awareness of need
	Appropriateness (goodness of provider-task match)
	Ability to initiate supportive efforts
	Knowledge of what is helpful
	Skills and experience
	Flexibility
	Adequacy of backup (relief available/alternate support givers)
Recipient	Prior support network status
	Ability to ask for help
	Current physical and emotional state (limitations on ability to accept help; change in support needs)
	Perceived need for support

(From Rowland,[61] with permission.)

continued support of the patient, it is also important to permit family members to limit care to those areas in which they are most comfortable and effective. For example, a spouse may be best equipped to provide affectional and nurturing support but may resist or be uncomfortable playing a decision-making role in questions of medical care or treatment, a task perhaps better suited to an adult son or daughter.

For their part, patients may not always welcome or correctly interpret the care extended by family (or by staff for that matter).[58] They may resist help because of concern about what others will think, cultural taboos associated with asking for help, or the sense of dependency and helplessness that such support engenders. The overly solicitous and jollying efforts of well-meaning spouses can make patients feel angry and isolated. When family members are expected to play an active role in specific rehabilitative tasks, it is necessary to explain to them how to go about doing so and to negotiate with the patients as to what is comfortable. Because patients' status, hence needs, change over time, periodic review of the type and level of support provided is essential. In working with patients who feel guilty about asking for or accepting assistance, it is helpful to emphasize that requests for aid make the spouse or family member feel useful in a time of crisis. Shifting perspective on help requests decreases patient concerns about being a burden and also serves to strengthen patients' sense that they can actively direct, not merely passively receive, aid.

Physical therapists need to consider all these issues when involving the family in rehabilitation plans and assigning tasks. When stress does occur in the system, they must look for and address the likely multiple etiologies of the dysfunction. Referral to another member of the treatment team (e.g., primary physician, social worker) for further action or follow-up may be appropriate. At times it may become apparent that the physical therapist is contributing to the problem.

Staff Stress

Providing physical therapy services to cancer patients can be highly stressful.[59] Sources of stress derive from three different levels: the nature of the work and the population being served; environmental demands; and personal characteristics of the therapist (see Table 7-4). Because of the nature of their disease, there is a high rate of morbidity and mortality among cancer patients. As a consequence, physical therapists working with this population must manage patients who are sicker than those with other ailments, who may have experienced multimodal therapy (surgery, radiotherapy, chemotherapy) resulting in multiple limitations and in some cases obvious disfigurement, and for whom prognosis is guarded. Although few physical therapists work solely with cancer patients, the increasing number of people being treated for, living with, and surviving cancer suggests that growing numbers will seek such services. Confrontation with issues of mortality and death are an expected part of this work. In addition, because many cancer patients are now followed over long periods,

Table 7-4. Sources of Staff Stress

Problem Areas	Issues
Nature of illness/patient population	High morbidity/high mortality Terminal care issues Potentially disfiguring treatments Aggressive multimodal therapy resulting in multiple side effects/ limits to full recovery Additional chronic illness in older patients
Health care environment	Complex technology/high pressure Demand for advanced training Multiple caregivers, resulting in increased opportunity for interstaff conflict/miscommunication Staff shortages Increased case load; decreased time Lack of staff support mechanisms Need to inflict pain as part of care

Personnel characteristics	Lack of or inability to access an effective support system
	Family tension; marital stress
	Multiple external problems/obligations
	Adverse reactions to patients
	    Separation/loss/grief
	    Overidentification/transference issues
	    Negative cancer attitudes/experience
	    Reluctance to work with subsets of patients (e.g., head and neck cancer)
	Need to see self as "healer"; high need for approval of patients/ staff

during which physical therapists may develop strong attachments to and observe progressive deterioration in special patients, risk for separation problems and distress over loss and death is increased. In order to tolerate the intense emotional demands of working with this population, a supportive work and social environment are critical, as are personal philosophy and resources. Nevertheless, there are multiple obstacles to achieving such a balance.

Increasing dependence on sophisticated technology in the provision of medical care has led to greater demands being made on staff with regard to training, time, and case load. Other work changes contributing to staff stress are staff shortages in certain areas (e.g., nursing); education that lags behind advances in biomedical applications; increased acuity of patients hospitalized and discharged home; the greater number of people involved in a given patient's care; and the decreased time allocated for care delivery despite augmented case loads. A common casualty of greater time demands is less time for support or time out for the health professional. The physical therapist's ability to tolerate such conditions depends in turn on a number of individual considerations.

As members of society, health care providers, like patients and their families, are exposed to the same beliefs and myths about cancer. Personal fears, anxieties, and misconceptions enter into caregiving practices and can adversely affect both provider performance and patient well-being. Sometimes this is overt, as in avoidance of particular patients; at other times the response may be revealed in nonverbal cues or in inconsistencies in behavior over time.[60] The characteristics of a patient may evoke strong transference reactions; an individual client may remind the therapist of a parent, sibling, child, close friend, or even of him- or herself, arousing disturbing emotions or previously unresolved conflicts that interfere with work. For therapists who entered the field dedicated to "helping" people, daily confrontation with progressive disease and feelings of ambivalence about the need to inflict pain in the course of their work may be demoralizing over time. Finally, the therapist's ability to cope with stressful demands may be compromised by lack of outside support. Examples include conflict at home, multiple external demands, or inability of friends and family to provide empathic understanding of and a buffer for the stressful nature of the physical therapist's work.

The first step in managing staff stress is to acknowledge that it is inherent in the type of work to be done and to identify the contribution made to it by the environment and the individual. More difficult are those situations in which members of the system fail or refuse to recognize that problems exist. Team meetings to discuss members' roles and review individual patient plans need to be regularly scheduled. Sessions involving only members of the physical therapy staff to discuss treatment problems and the more general issues of working with cancer patients are helpful. These sessions need not be formal. Another function they serve is to monitor staff well-being and provide a mutual support system. Staff who work primarily with cancer patients often find themselves stigmatized in social settings (i.e., few people want to hear about their work). Thus, development of alternative sources of personal support and validation for their role is important.

By way of caring for oneself, it is important to schedule time away for enjoyable activities to offset the expected stress of caring for cancer patients and occasional periods of frustration. Requesting additional help and/or informing supervisors about needed schedule or work load changes during particularly stressful periods at home or work can help reduce feelings of burnout. Of equal importance is the need to be sensitive to one's own reactions to working in physical therapy. It is clear that some individuals are more comfortable than others in working with specific patient populations (e.g., burn victims, facially disfigured patients). At times, achieving a sense of comfort is a question of time and experience. In other cases the resistance may be deep-seated. When conflict arises around this issue, referral to a counselor may be appropriate. It should also be recognized that there are some patients whom nobody likes. The hateful patient presents a particularly difficult challenge for the health professional. When working with these individuals, it is useful to share responsibility with other staff members and to remind oneself that the belief that one has to be able to work well with everyone is just a belief, not an expectation.

Perhaps the greatest stress buffer of all is the therapy work itself. With the majority of cancer patients, the physical therapist can observe and measure improvement over time, sometimes even when the oncologist has been able only to arrest temporarily or stabilize the disease. The satisfaction and joys of returned function are celebrated by all—patient, family, and staff alike. Even when care is palliative, physical therapists can feel that they are integrally involved in enhancing quality of survival for patients. Indeed, use of physical therapy with advanced cancer patients often serves to provide hope and a sense of continued self-worth and meaning to the patient.

SUMMARY

As increasing numbers of cancer patients are surviving and being cured of their disease, the importance of rehabilitation, and in particular of the role played by physical therapists, is growing. Disease, patient, social, and staff variables all affect the patient's ability to actively participate in rehabilitative efforts and achieve full recovery. Knowledge of these and of their implications for patient management in physical therapy is important. Because of the nature of their involvement with patients, physical therapists are uniquely situated to identify and help address areas of patient distress, and in this role they serve to promote not only optimal physical well-being but also psychological recovery of patients, which makes them vital participants in the treatment team.

REFERENCES

1. Holland JC: Clinical course of cancer. p. 75. In Holland JC, Rowland JH (eds): Handbook of Psychooncology: Psychological Care of the Patient with Cancer. Oxford University Press, New York, 1989
2. Holland JC, Rowland J, Lebovitz A, Rusalem R: Reactions to cancer treatment: Assessment of emotional response to adjuvant radiotherapy as a guide to planned intervention. Psychiatr Clin North Am 2:347, 1979
3. Dietz JH Jr: Rehabilitation of the cancer patient: Its role in the scheme of comprehensive care. Clin Bull 4:104, 1974
4. DeLisa JA, Miller RM, Melnick RR et al: Rehabilitation of the cancer patient. p. 2333. In DeVita VT, Rosenberg SA, Hellman S (eds): Cancer: Principles and Practice of Oncology 3rd Ed. JB Lippincott, Philadelphia, 1989
5. Harvey RF, Jellinek HM, Habeck RV: Cancer rehabilitation: An analysis of 36 program approaches. JAMA 247:2127, 1982
6. Hamburg DA, Adams JE: A perspective on coping behavior: Seeking and utilizing information in major transition. Arch Gen Psychiatry 17:277, 1967
7. Weisman D: Early diagnosis of vulnerability in cancer patients. Am J Med Sci 271:187, 1976
8. Penman DT: Coping strategies in adaptation to mastectomy. Psychosom Med 44:117, 1982
9. Thoits PA: Social support as coping assistance. J Consult Clin Psychol 54:416, 1986
10. Cohen S, Syme SL (eds): Social Support and Health. Academic Press, Orlando, FL, 1985
11. Dunkel-Schetter C: Social support and cancer: Findings based on patient interviews and their implications. J Soc Issues 40:77, 1984
12. Morrow GR, Hoagland AC: Physician-patient communication in cancer treatment. p. 27. In Proceedings American Cancer Society, 3rd National Conference on Human Values and Cancer. Washington, April 23–25, 1981

13. Hoffman B: Cancer survivors at work: Job problems and illegal discrimination. Oncol Nurs Forum 16:39, 1989
14. Feldman FL: Work and cancer health histories. American Cancer Society, California Division, San Francisco, 1982
15. Breitbart W, Holland JC: Head and neck cancer. p. 232. In Holland JC, Rowland JH (eds): Handbook of Psychooncology: Psychological Care of the Patient with Cancer. Oxford University Press, New York, 1989
16. Shedd DR: Cancer of the head and neck. p. 167. In Holland JF, Frei E III (eds): Cancer Medicine. 2nd Ed. Lea & Febiger, Philadelphia, 1982
17. Dropkin MJ, Malgady RG, Scott DW, et al: Scaling of disfigurement and dysfunction in postoperative head and neck patients. Head Neck Surg 8:559, 1983
18. Natvig K: Social, personal and behavioral factors related to present mastery of the laryngectomy event. J Otolaryngol 12:155, 1983
19. Goldberg RT: Vocational and social adjustment after laryngectomy. Scand J Rehabil Med 7:1, 1975
20. West DW: Social adaptation patterns among cancer patients with facial disfigurements resulting from surgery. Arch Phys Med Rehabil 58:473, 1977
21. Holland JC: Lung Cancer. p. 180. In Holland JC, Rowland JH (eds): Handbook of Psychooncology: Psychological Care of the Patient with Cancer. Oxford University Press, New York, 1989
22. Cancer Facts and Figures—1989. American Cancer Society, Atlanta, 1989
23. Hughes JE: Depressive illness and lung cancer: I. Depression before diagnosis. Eur J Surg Oncol 11:15, 1985
24. Minna JD, Pass H, Glatstein E, Inde DC: Cancer of the lung. p. 591. In DeVita VT, Hellman S, Rosenberg SA (eds): Cancer: Principles and Practice of Oncology. 3rd Ed. JB Lippincott, Philadelphia, 1989
25. Johnson BE, Goff WB II, Petronas MA, et al: Neurologic, neuropsychologic and computed cranial tomography scan abnormalities in 2- to 10-year survivors of small-cell lung cancer. J Clin Oncol 3: 1659, 1985
26. Driever MJ, McCorkle R: Patient concerns at 3 and 6 months postdiagnosis. Cancer Nurs 7:235, 1984
27. Yates JW, Chalmer B, McKegney FP: Evaluation of patients with advanced cancer using the Karnofsky performance status. Cancer 40:2220, 1980
28. Cella DF, Orofiamma B, Holland JC et al: The relationship of psychological distress, extent of disease, and performance status in patients with lung cancer. Cancer 60:1661, 1987
29. Trillin AS: Of dragons and garden peas: A cancer patient talks to doctors. N Engl J Med 304:699, 1981
30. Mack RM: Occasional notes: Lessons from living with cancer. N Engl J Med 311:1640, 1984
31. Meyerowitz BE: Psychosocial correlates of breast cancer and its treatment. Psychol Bull 87:108, 1980
32. Bloom J, Cook M, Fotopoulis S et al: Psychological response to mastectomy: A prospective comparison study. Cancer 59:189, 1987
33. Ashcroft JJ, Leinster SJ, Slade PD: Breast cancer—patient choice of treatment: Preliminary communication. J R Soc Med 78:43, 1985
34. Margolis GJ, Goodman RL: Psychological factors in women choosing radiation therapy for breast cancer. Psychosomatics 25:464, 1984
35. Holland JC, Rowland JH: Psychological reactions to breast cancer and its treatment. p. 632. In Harris JR, Hellman S, Henderson IC, Kinne DW (eds): Breast Diseases. JB Lippincott, Philadelphia, 1987

36. Wellisch DK, DiMatteo R, Silverstein M, et al.: Psychosocial outcomes of breast cancer therapies: Lumpectomy versus mastectomy. Psychosomatics 30:365, 1989 Psychosomatics (in press)

37. Zevon MA, Rounds JB, Karr J: Psychological outcomes associated with breast conserving surgery: A meta-analysis. Presented at 8th annual meeting of the Society of Behavioral Medicine, Washington, March 1987

38. Euster S: Rehabilitation after mastectomy: The group process. Soc Work Health Care 4:251, 1979

39. Wellisch DK, Jamison, KR, Pasnau O: Psychosocial aspects of mastectomy. II. The man's perspective. Am J Psychiatry 135:543, 1978

40. Holland JC, Massie MJ: Psychosocial aspects of cancer in the elderly. Clin Geriatr Med 3:533,1987

41. Cassileth BR, Lusk EJ, Strouse TB, et al: Psychosocial status in chronic illness: A comparative analysis of six diagnostic groups. N Engl J Med 311:506, 1984

42. Maisiak R, Gams R, Lee E, Jones B: The psychosocial support status of elderly cancer outpatients. Prog Clin Biol Res 120:395, 1983

43. Ganz PA, Schag CC, Heinrich RL: The psychosocial impact of cancer on the elderly: A comparison with younger patients. J Am Geriatr Soc 33:429, 1985

44. Bloom J, Gorsky R, Fobair P, et al: Changes in the physical performance in men following treatment for Hodgkin's disease. Proc Am Soc Clin Oncol 6:258 (Abstract No. 1016), 1987

45. Smith SD, Rosen D, Trueworthy RC, Lowman JT: A reliable method for evaluating drug compliance in children with cancer. Cancer 43:169, 1979

46. Mather L, Mackie J: The incidence of postoperative pain in children. Pain 15:271, 1983

47. Bush JP: Pain in children: A review of the literature from a developmental perspective. Psychol Health 1:215, 1987

48. Kagan LB: Use of denial in adolescents with bone cancer. Health Soc Work 1:71, 1976

49. Sugarbaker PH, Barofsky I, Rosenberg SA, Gianola FJ: Quality of life assessment of patients in extremity sarcoma trials. Surgery 91:17, 1982

50. Boyle M, Tebbi CK, Mindell ER, Mettlin LJ: Adolescent adjustment to amputation. Med Pediatr Oncol 10:301, 1982

51. Weddington WW, Seagraves KB, Simon MA: Psychological outcome of extremity sarcoma survivors undergoing amputation or limb salvage. J Clin Oncol 3:1393, 1985

52. Auchincloss SS: Sexual dysfunction in cancer patients: Issues in evaluation and treatment. p. 383. In Holland JC, Rowland JH (eds): Handbook of Psychooncology: Psychological Care of the Patient with Cancer. Oxford University Press, New York, 1989

53. Vincent CE, Vincent FC, Greiss FC, Linton EB: Some marital-sexual concomitants of carcinoma of the cervix. South Med J 68:552, 1975

54. Schover LR, Jensen SB: Sexuality and Chronic Illness: A Comprehensive Approach. Guilford Press, New York, 1988

55. Vaeth JM (ed): Body Image, Self-Esteem, and Sexuality in Cancer Patients. 2nd Ed. Karger, Basel, Switzerland, 1986

56. Wortman CB: Social support and the cancer patient: Conceptual and methodologic issues. Cancer 53:2339, 1984

57. Rait D, Lederberg M: The family of the cancer patient. p. 585. In Holland JC, Rowland JH (eds): Handbook of Psychooncology: Psychological Care of the Patient with Cancer. Oxford University Press, New York, 1989

58. Fisher JD, Nadler A, Whitcher-Alagna S: Recipient reactions to aid. Psychol Bull 91:27, 1982
59. Lederberg MS: Psychological problems of staff and their management. p. 631. In Holland JC, Rowland JH (eds): Handbook of Psychooncology: Psychological Care of the Patient with Cancer. Oxford University Press, New York, 1989
60. Dunkel-Schetter C, Wortman C: The interpersonal dynamics of cancer: Problems in social relationships and their impact on the patient. p. 69. In Friedman HS, DiMatteo MR (eds): Interpersonal Issues in Health Care. Academic Press, Orlando, FL, 1982
61. Rowland JH: Interpersonal resources: Social support. p. 67. In Holland JC, Rowland JII (eds.). Handbook of Psychooncology: Psychological Care of the Patient with Cancer. Oxford University Press, New York, 1989

8 | Care of the Terminally Ill: Hospice, Home, and Extended Care Facilities

Rick Reuss
Sharon Last

Since the late 1950s there has been an explosion of information available in the medical community on the subject of death and dying. Dr. Elisabeth Kubler-Ross is acknowledged as one of the pioneers in the United States in dealing with this formerly taboo subject. She has introduced the concept of five stages of dying: denial and isolation, anger, bargaining, depression, and acceptance. She and subsequently many other writers and medical practitioners have provided the general public, as well as the medical community, with a wealth of information and insight into the introspective and, hopefully, extrospective aspects of one's own mortality and ways of responding to this challenging and inevitable life event.

Since the early 1960s Drs. Cicely Saunders and Richard Lamerton have contributed immeasurably to the field of medicine by delineating the multifaceted hospice approach to the care of terminally ill people in England. This approach has now enjoyed attention and practical application in many different settings and facilities in the United States, which has led to a proliferation of medical literature regarding it, but this literature has been primarily directed to the physician and nurse.

It has been only since the late 1970s that articles specifically dealing with the involvement of physical therapy in the care of the terminally ill patient, most often the terminally ill cancer patient, have been published nationally.

THE PHASES OF CANCER TREATMENT

As has been noted quite admirably in the preceding pages of this book, the curative phase of cancer intervention primarily consists of the new and innovative treatment approaches of chemotherapy, immunotherapy, radiotherapy, and surgery.

The palliative phase of cancer treatment is broadly noted in terms of palliative chemotherapy for management of systemic metastases to alleviate visceral symptoms; palliative radiotherapy of specific organ metastases or bone and brain metastases; palliative pharmacologic and chemical intervention to control pain and other manifestations of metastasis; and palliative surgical intervention directed to space-occupying or life-threatening metastases. The palliative phase is directed toward new areas of metastases or involvement of body systems secondary to the curative measures taken.

In many instances the palliative phase concludes with the terminal phase of cancer treatment, when the disease has progressed to the point at which curative and restorative treatment is no longer a reasonable goal and prolonging life is no longer the objective of medical care.

The time that a cancer patient spends in transition from the curative to the palliative to the terminal phase may last from days or weeks to years. With appropriate training in the physiologic and psychological implications of the dying process, the process of grief, and a sound philosophy of the care of the dying patient, the physical therapist can be well equipped to provide valuable assistance to the cancer patient. This can be accomplished, not only in the curative phase but also in the palliative and finally the terminal phase of care, through the use of physical therapy skills.

It is generally accepted that the hospice concept of care serves as the appropriate medical model for all disciplines in assisting cancer patients with their transition from curative through palliative to the terminal phases of their disease. It is acknowledged that there is currently debate in both the medical and secular communities over the merits of passive euthanasia (i.e., voluntary withholding of medical treatment and thereby hastening the death process).[1] The arguments for euthanasia, active or passive, societally condoned suicide, or any intervention in the name of medicine to hasten the patient's death conflict with the basic philosophy of hospice care.

The National Hospice Organization defines *hospice* as a centrally administered program of palliative and supportive services, which provides physical, psychological, social, and spiritual care for dying patients and their families. Services are provided by a medically supervised interdisciplinary team of professionals and volunteers. Hospice services are available in both a home and an inpatient setting. Home care is provided on a part-time, intermittent, regularly scheduled, around-the-clock, on-call basis. Bereavement services are also available to the family. Admission to a hospice program is on the basis of patient and family need.

The goal of hospice intervention is to affirm and promote the quality of life until death, not to prolong life through extraordinary means. A primary objective is to keep the patient pain-free but alert so that the patient and family will have the opportunity to achieve a level of satisfactory mental and spiritual preparation for death.

Hospice intervention has three main focuses, which distinguish this concept from the traditional medical model of health care. The primary objective is to assist the patient to remain home as long as possible, ideally until death. Second, inpatient care is provided in a hospital or other inpatient facility should the patient no longer be able to remain at home or the family no longer be able to cope with the patient at home. Finally, bereavement services provide guidance in preparation for the patient's death and follow-up support for the family after the death for as long as the support is necessary. The patient and the immediate family not just the patient, are considered the primary unit of care.

It is generally understood that there are currently few physical therapists practicing in formal hospice settings; however, the principles of hospice care, particularly with regard to the role of the physical therapist, can be used by physical therapists in any practice setting where patients are encountered who have made the transition from the curative to the palliative phase of treatment and ultimately to the terminal phase of their disease process. The hospice model is predicated on the multidisciplinary approach to patient care, with which all physical therapists are well acquainted.

THE INTERDISCIPLINARY TEAM

An intermingling of roles is inherent in the hospice concept of care, in that the team members of the hospice not only know their specific roles but also draw upon resources from other team members. Great importance is placed on when to ask for that assistance or intervention by other team members. The basic interdisciplinary hospice team consists of the chaplain, the nurse, the pharmacist, the physician, the volunteer, and the physical therapist. Consultants to the core hospice team include a host of other professionals: clinical psychologist, clinical psychiatrist, dietician, funeral director, general surgeon, home health aide, medical oncologist, neurosurgeon, occupational therapist, oncologic radiotherapist, plastic surgeon, and speech pathologist. The most important member of the team, of course, is the patient, who along with the family guides and monitors the success of all plans of intervention.

The Chaplain

One of the current ongoing challenges of hospice programs is to delineate ways of providing meaningful spiritual and religious support for patients and their families while still respecting the privacy of the family unit. The basic responsibility of the chaplain is to be available for spiritual, religious, and philosophical guidance to the patient and family and to coordinate community pastoral care services. The chaplain also serves as an ethical consultant to the interdisciplinary team and counselor for the spiritual concerns of the staff members.

The Nurse

One of the integral components of the hospice concept is staffing by nurses skilled in pain management and symptom control. Nursing services help keep team members apprised of patient physical and psychological changes or new developments in the patient's medical condition. Direct nursing services generally include routine visits; patient assessment to determine health care needs; identification of alterations in health status of patient; initiation of a plan of individual nursing care; and participation in the on-call schedule to meet the emergency needs of the patient.

Since the late 1970s there seems to be a movement away from the model of a central hospice team to that of "hospice" services provided by neighborhood visiting nurse organizations, with consultation by nurses with other practitioners on a case by case basis. Further, there seems to be confusion in some nursing communities, as demonstrated by the premise that if one takes care of terminally ill patients, one is providing "hospice" services, albeit without specific training in the tenets of hospice care, particularly in home health settings. Practitioners must understand the difference between care given through recognized hospice programs and quasi-hospice components of health care agencies.

The Pharmacist

One of the most important reasons why the hospice concept of care has enjoyed success in the treatment of the terminal cancer patient has been its emphasis on successful pain intervention. The pharmacist, as a team member, ensures that pain control is successful by providing the necessary expertise to enable the health care team to understand the basic concepts of clinical pharmacology.

The pharmacist is responsible for patient and family consultation in ensuring an adequate daily drug supply to alleviate not only pain but also the other common symptoms of constipation, depression, and nausea, and vomiting. In concert with the team, the pharmacist maintains drug profile monitoring, provides individual dosage titration for analgesic use for resolution of chronic cancer pain, and displays proficiency in the use of equianalgesic charts.

The Physician

The hospice physician is the primary consultant in the team care effort, through whom all physical care efforts are coordinated. The direct services of the hospice physician include patient visits and assessments to determine appropriate pain and symptom intervention; clarification of the dying process to the patient and family; referral of patient care needs to appropriate team members; assumption of responsibility for regulation of appropriate medicines; provision of comprehensive physical and psychological care of the patient and family; and collaboration and liaison with attending physicians.

The Social Worker

The social worker in the hospice concept of care provides individual, marital, and family counseling and assists with financial concerns as well as serving as a coordinator of community resources. The value of the social worker to the patient, patient's family, and team can be seen in social crisis intervention; improvement in the method and mode of communication; helping the family to work as a unit in confronting the process of terminal illness and bereavement; and facilitation of appropriate team dynamics.

The Volunteer

Hospice volunteers are a particularly special group of people. They are generally selected through established recruitment procedures and are trained in the hospice concept of care.

Volunteer services run the gamut of direct patient and family assistance. Volunteers provide nontechnical bedside care (bathing, lifting, feeding, dressing, etc); run errands; provide personal support and companionship; are available at the time of death if a family member cannot be present; provide an atmosphere of warmth and understanding for the family; and assist in bereavement follow-up with the family after the patient's death.

Role of Physical Therapy

The hospice physical therapist is responsible for assisting patients in all areas of mobility, modified exercise programs, bed positioning, and arranging for equipment at the patient's home to minimize effort and assist in pain control.

The job description and protocol for intervention given in Appendices 1 and 2, respectively, are applicable to any practice setting involving the terminal cancer patient. These policies were developed for an operating hospice program.

SYMPTOM CONTROL
Pain Control

One of the main reasons for referring a patient for hospice care is to provide alleviation of physical pain. Pain control in most instances is accomplished by the around-the-clock administration of narcotic pain medication. The medication is administered by the patient, a family member, a caregiver, or an external medication device. The main point is that the patient should receive the precise amount of medication necessary to alleviate the pain. This process is generally accomplished within a few days of the beginning of hospice care.

The physical therapist may be included in the initial assessment visit but most often receives referral on the occasion when the patient's pain is at a satisfactory level to allow participation in normal daily activities. Addiction to the prescribed around-the-clock pain medication is not an issue unless the medication is withheld. The therapist must also continue to be cognizant of the symptoms of constipation, which follows administration of narcotic pain medication. These symptoms may affect the patient's ability to perform the therapeutic program comfortably.

Symptoms of Dying

In participating in the care of the terminal cancer patient, the physical therapist must know the general pattern of events preceding the actual death. Patients become more somnolent and diaphoretic. Although anoxia is a classic symptom of chemotherapy and cancer, one cardinal rule understood by experienced hospice team members involves eating and drinking behaviors. If patients stop eating, death may be a week or so away, and if they stop drinking fluids, death may be a few days away. Pain medication can be satisfactorily reduced in response to the patient's request, as the physical pain is generally reduced at the end of life. Patients respond less to family members and their environment, their eyes turn up and roll back, and their fingers and toes become cyanotic. It is at this time that family members, as well as medical caregivers, need to say their goodbyes.

The actual dying process and the event of death should be communicated honestly and appropriately to the family members. The actual death of hospice patients is generally quiet and peaceful to the point where those family members in attendance may wait for a time before informing the hospice program and calling the funeral home.

FEARS OF THE TERMINALLY ILL

The fears most frequently identified with dying include fears of pain; of progressive deterioration and disability; of loss of control over personal decisions; of being left alone; of overwhelming emotional feelings; of not knowing what is happening; of being buried alive; and of receiving inadequate medical care.[1] Through the successful intervention of the hospice program, most of the patient's and family's fears surrounding death are alleviated sufficiently that they can continue with the life process until the time of the patient's death. From alleviation of fear comes hope. Purtilo has said[2]:

That the patient will almost always find something to still hope for is the most important thing the therapist should remember.. . . The physical therapist can best help the person find meaning in the experience of physical disability or terminal illness by listening to and taking seriously these expressed hopes. The therapist cannot always promise that the hopes will be fulfilled, but he or she can always assure the patient that the hopes have been heard. The therapist, also, can often play a significant role in helping the person to realize one or more of the hopes by something as simple as a phone call or change in treatment.

DISCUSSION

Unlike hospices in Europe, which were primarily founded and led by physicians, the majority of U.S. hospice programs are coordinated by nurses. Neither discipline has a monopoly on leadership in this concept of care. In fact, the House of Delegates of the American Physical Therapy Association in 1978 passed a resolution supporting the position that it is the right and responsibility of each health care facility to select the individual health professional best qualified by education, experience, and unique individual leadership character-istics to coordinate all physician-prescribed care, or any portion thereof, and care delivered in that facility by nonphysician health personnel. Physical thera-pists have an obligation not only to participate in the care of the terminally ill, but also to assume leadership positions in such programs should the opportuni-ties to serve in this way arise.

For a physical therapist, participation in the care of terminal cancer patients can be one of the most satisfying and fulfilling experiences in a professional career. One reaches the point at which one accepts the miraculous and condones the commonplace. The heroics that go on and the internal dynamics within families are incredible. They (the family members and the patient) affirm so clearly that which is right and good, allowing one to "see then" the "games" that go on with so many contemporary peers or patients. There is a general honesty that pervades almost every interaction.

The therapy (e.g., exercise, walking, or pain modality) either works or does not work. There is no time for the strategy of "it might work," as it is necessary to proceed with solving specific problems. Generally, if the solution is available, one arrives at what is physically possible or acknowledges and accepts what is physically impossible. The importance of being "allowed to fail," even when life is waning, can be a critical event for the individual therapist. What is part of life must be allowed at death. Either as the physical therapist or as a patient with a limited life expectancy, one must be allowed to fail and in that failure affirm what is true and good.

CONCLUSION

Participation in the care of terminally ill patients generally affirms what Faulkner said[3]:

I believe that man will not merely endure, but that he will prevail. Man is immortal not only because he alone among all creatures has an inexhaustible voice, but because he has a soul, a spirit capable of compassion and sacrifice and endurance.

The physical therapist is an essential person in the care of the terminal cancer patient. Within that role is the reminder of the therapist's own mortality, as only through this realization can one effectively assist others in dealing with their own finiteness or imminent death. Stewart Alsop, while contemplating his own condition of acute myeloblastic leukemia, said[4]:

Death is, after all, the only universal experience except birth, and although a sensible person hopes to put it off as long as possible, it is, even in anticipation, an interesting experience.

REFERENCES

1. Wanzer SH, Federman DD, Adelstein SJ, et al: The physician's responsibility toward hopelessly ill patients: A second look. N Engl J Med 320:844, 1989
2. Worden JW, Proctor W: P.D.A./Personal Death Awareness—Breaking Free of Fear to Live a Better Life Now. Prentice-Hall, Englewood Cliffs, NJ, 1976, pp. 51–66
3. Purtilo RB: Similarities in patient response to chronic and terminal illness. Phys Ther 56(3):283, 1976
4. Faulkner W: Formal essay (upon his receipt of Nobel Prize), Stockholm, Sweden, 1950
5. Alsop S: Stay of Execution. JB Lippincott, Philadelphia, 1973

SUGGESTED READINGS

Buckingham RW, Lack SA, Mount BM, et al: Living with the dying: Use of the technique of participant observation. Can Med Assoc J 115:1211, 1975

Cammack JM: Interdisciplinary care of the patient with cancer in a community hospital. Clin Management Phys Ther 2(4):7, 1982

Davis CM: Hospice care: Physical therapy has a role to play. Clin Management Phys Ther 2(2):7, 1982

Downie PA: Rehabilitation of the cancer patient. Nurs Mirror Sep 29:36, 1972

Lamerton R: Care of the Dying. Technomic Publishing, Westport CT, 1976

Purtilo RB: Similarities in patient response to chronic and terminal illness. Phys Ther 56:279, 1976

Purtilo RB: Health Professional/Patient Interaction. 2nd Ed, WB Saunders, Philadelphia, 1978

Purtilo RB, Cassel CK: Ethnical Dimensions in the Health Professions. WB Saunders, Philadelphia, 1981

Reuss R: Hospice: One PT's personal account. Clin Management Phys Ther 4(6):28, 1984

Reuss, R: The use of TENS in the management of cancer pain. Clin Management Phys Ther 5(5):26, 1985

Saunders, C: A death in the family: A professional view. Br Med J 1:31, 1973

Shanks R: Physiotherapy in palliative care. Physiotherapy 68:405, 1982

Shephard, DAE: Principles and practice of palliative care. Can Med Assoc J 116:522, 1977

Tillett W: The role of a physiotherapist in a hospice. NZ J Physiother 10(2):20, 1982

Toot J: Physical therapy and hospice: Concept and practice. Phys Ther 64:665, 1984

Will G: A good death. Indiana Med 71:734, 1978

Worden JW, Proctor W: P.D.A./Personal Death Awareness-Breaking Free of Fear to Live a Better Life Now. Prentice-Hall, Englewood Cliffs, NJ, 1976

Appendices

Prerequisites

Physical therapy services, when provided, are given by a licensed physical therapist or by a licensed physical therapist assistant under the supervision of a licensed physical therapist in accordance with a plan of treatment.

Definition of Services

Direct services (patient/family oriented)

1. Examination and documentation of functional abilities and deficits
2. Instruction of patient in the appropriate mode of ambulation or functional mobility
3. Administration of relevant exercise that may be necessary for performance of activities of daily living
4. Identification of realistic functional goals with patient and family
5. Administration of palliative modalities for adjunctive relief of pain
6. Implementation of all necessary precautions for the proper care and safety of patient
7. Instruction of patient and family in proper body mechanics
8. Home evaluation to determine accessibility of patient's domicile

Indirect services

1. Attendance at all patient care meetings
2. Discussion of patient treatment, care, and progress with hospice medical director and appropriate hospice team members
3. Instruction of all hospice team members in proper body mechanics
4. Participation in continuing education of the medical and civic community in the hospice concept
5. Writing or collaboration in writing professional articles concerned with hospice care
6. Participation in quality assessment program developed and implemented by the hospice program

Appendix 8-2. Physical Therapy Protocol: Terminally Ill Patient Admitted to Hospice

Criteria for referral (one of the following is sufficient)
1. Patients with obvious preexisting or concurrent physical disabilities, which may limit mobility or functional activities
2. Patients determined by the hospice medical director or other hospice team members to require adjunctive pain relief through application of transcutaneous electrical nerve stimulation (TENS) or other physical modalities
3. Patients and/or families who identify problems at place of patient residence in the areas of architectural barriers precluding mobility; motor dysfunction presenting difficulty in mobility or locomotion (e.g., bed mobility, toilet transfers, ambulation); and patient lifting
4. Patients who have been bedfast for an appreciable length of time
5. Patients currently in hospice program who have sustained physical complications causing dramatic decline in physical function
6. Refusal of family to assist patient in functional activities of daily living
7. Identified need for discharge planning of physical needs and patient/family training for in-hospital or extended care facility patients

Protocol for physical therapy intervention
    Assessment
        Process
1. Referral
2. Review of previous or current medical chart and/or oncology chart
3. Initial evaluation of patient (as indicated and tolerated)
    a) Recognition of areas in which structure and function are abnormal
    b) Specification of which physical therapy assessment procedures are indicated
    c) Performance of definitive physical therapy testing of neurologic, skeletal, muscular, and cardiovascular systems
    d) Assessment of patient environment from focus of architectural barriers to mobility and modifications required for simplification of patient activities of daily living
        Information to be obtained
1. Pertinent past medical/physical history as related to function and mobility
2. Patient and family response to present terminal condition and previous response to debilitating illness
3. Specific physical difficulties encountered by patient and family
4. Present level of patient physical and functional ability
5. Patient and family expectations of physical potential for mobility and function
6. Available resources
    a) Family members and significant others to physically assist patient
    b) Outside agencies to assist with procurement of assistive equipment
    Goal setting and implementation of plan
1. Design and management of a physical therapy plan of care meeting the following requirements:
    a) Realistic goals in terms of physical/mental status and life-style of patient. Goals established with patient, family, medical director, and relevant hospice team members
    b) Methods that provide a high probability of achieving goals
    c) Engagement of the greatest possible degree of patient and family motivation and cooperation
    d) Within resource constraints;
    e) Provision for periodic revision
    f) Provision for quality assessment
    g) Provision for maximum goal achievement with minimal energy and time expenditure
    h) Safety for the patient, family, and caregivers
    i) Based on empirical/scientific rationale
    j) Specificity and comprehensiveness appropriate to the level of personnel who will execute the plan
    k) Adequate documentation

(continued)

Appendix 8-2. Physical Therapy Protocol: Terminally Ill Patient Admitted to Hospice (*continued*)

2. Implementation of a specific physical therapy plan of care that includes the direct or delegated application of the following modalities:
   a) Physical agents (ice packs, warms soaks, massage, TENS, etc)
   b) Gait training
   c) Assistive equipment/ambulatory aides
   d) Functional activities and exercises
   e) Work simplification
   f) Therapeutic equipment
3. Modification of physical therapy goals or plan
4. Evaluation and interpretation of and response to changes in the physiologic/mental state of patient
5. Identification of and recommendations regarding architectural barriers that
   a) Provide optimal solutions of the problems
   b) Do not create unmanageable barriers for others
   c) Are acceptable to the patient and family
   d) Are safe
   e) Are appropriate to the patient's terminal prognosis
   f) Are within resource constraints
   g) Are adequately documented
6. Interaction with patients and families in a manner that provides the desired psychosocial support
   a) Recognition by physical therapists of their own reaction to death and dying
   b) Recognition of patients' and families' reactions to death and dying
   c) Respect for individual, cultural, religious, and socioeconomic differences
   d) Use of appropriate communication processes
7. Demonstration of appropriate and effective written, verbal, and nonverbal communication with patients and their families, colleagues, and the public
8. Demonstration of safe, ethical, and legal practice
9. Participation in a quality assessment program

Recording
1. Summary of assessment and treatment plan (i.e., method of implementation) noted in patient medical chart
2. Summary of intervention (i.e., progress toward specific goals or resolution of major problem) documented in chart

Unexpected events that interfere with implementation of physical therapy plan of care
1. Patient/family refusal of service
2. Patient withdrawal from hospice program
3. Unwillingness of patient and/or family to cooperate
4. Patient in a physical condition that precludes physical therapy intervention

Criteria for termination of physical therapy services
1. Goals of physical therapy intervention achieved
2. Death, unless bereavement follow-up indicated by physical therapist
3. Patient refusal of physical therapy intervention
4. Impossibility of achieving goals

9 | Research in Cancer Rehabilitation

Carolyn Cook Gotay

IMPORTANCE AND CURRENT STATUS OF CANCER REHABILITATION RESEARCH

Research has a number of important roles to play in cancer rehabilitation. Identifying and measuring rehabilitation problems is a critical first step in treatment, which relies upon assessment instruments that have been found to be valid, reliable, and clinically useful. Selecting optimal treatment regimens, including ascertaining the merits of new approaches, choosing among available alternatives, and making modifications to existing protocols, relies on the findings of rigorous research. Extending the scope of rehabilitation beyond the individual patient requires programmatic research on the effectiveness of rehabilitation strategies within the context of health care as a whole, including outcomes such as the cost-effectiveness and long-term impact of rehabilitation on the physical, psychosocial, and vocational-economic well-being of the patient and family.

Despite its importance, the current status of cancer rehabilitation research reflects a number of problems. For one, little research on cancer patients is being reported by the rehabilitation community. For example, reviews of abstracts submitted to the annual meetings of two organizations that are pacesetters in the field of rehabilitation research, the American Academy of Physical Medicine and Rehabilitation and the American Congress of Rehabilitation Medicine, were conducted for the 1972 to 1976[1] and 1982 to 1986 periods.[1,2] The proportion of abstracts that related to cancer was 1.6 percent in the earlier time interval and 2.6 in the latter despite a more than twofold increase in the total number of abstracts in the later time period.

This lack of emphasis on cancer rehabilitation is reflected in federal research funding as well. The major federal support for cancer research in the United States comes from the National Cancer Institute (NCI), which is part of the National Institutes of Health. An analysis of support (both cancer control and regular research grants) in NCI's Division of Cancer Prevention and Control, which administers the majority of the institute's rehabilitation projects, showed that about $3.3 million of a total of $108.3 million went for cancer rehabilitation research.[2]

An analysis of the kinds of ongoing cancer rehabilitation research was conducted by Gotay and Yates,[2] who examined the state of this research field as reflected in three sources: the 40 cancer-specific abstracts presented at the 1982 to 1986 rehabilitation meetings cited above; the literature (as shown in a Medline review using the constraints *cancer* and *rehabilitation* for the years 1980 to 1986, which yielded 108 articles); and NCI support (based on awards made in fiscal 1986).

Head and neck cancer emerged as a leading research topic in all three sources. Among the cancer-specific abstracts, 15 percent related to head and neck cancer patients (a proportion exceeded only by the area of amputee research, which accounted for 23 percent of the total abstracts). The major focus for both the literature and NCI funding was also head and neck cancer; 44 percent of articles and 42 percent of NCI funding related to such patients. It is heartening to note that head and neck cancer, which presents multifaceted rehabilitation challenges, is receiving research attention. At the same time it should be recognized that head and neck cancer patients represent only a small proportion of all cancer patients seen by rehabilitation specialists. The relative under-representation of research on frequent rehabilitation problems illustrates one of the gaps in the rehabilitation research literature as it now stands.

OBSTACLES TO CANCER
REHABILITATION RESEARCH

There are a number of reasons why cancer rehabilitation research may be undersupported, both within the cancer rehabilitation community and by external agencies. While some of the problems in this research area reflect general difficulties,[3] cancer rehabilitation poses its own set of distinctive challenges.

The Heterogeneity of Cancer and Its Treatment

A wide variety of diseases and treatments are included within the label *cancer*, which complicates the identification of the appropriate population for research. Cancer patients differ in site of disease, stage of disease, type of therapy, kinds of rehabilitation needs, and functional ability, as well as in many other individual characteristics that have implications for rehabilitation. Too often, research (especially in the psychosocial rehabilitation area) has tended to amalgamate responses based on "cancer patients" as a whole without considering how the specifics of the disease and treatment may influence research findings; thus, the interpretability of this research has been ambiguous. The nature of the disease and of the treatment have implications for the choice of study population, control groups, stratification, and analytic strategies. However, as the researcher limits the patient population to control for all these factors, it becomes increasingly difficult to enroll sufficient numbers of patients to provide answers to research questions within a finite time.

The Progressive Nature of the Disease

Overall, one-half of newly diagnosed cancer patients will succumb to their disease. Over a period of many years when the disease alternately exacerbates and remits, conventional rehabilitation approaches used in dealing with a fixed deficit are often questionable. Cancer rehabilitation therapy must be flexible enough to incorporate frequent reassessments and modifications to rehabilitation protocols in response to disease progression. A variety of rehabilitation goals are also possible at a given time—restoration, support, and palliation.[4] Because of the nature of the disease, research in this area can sometimes seem to be like ''chasing a moving target.'' Research designs that incorporate multiple times of measurement are often the best choices to assess changes in functioning over time. However, missing data and patient attrition make this kind of research particularly difficult.

While cancer is an ultimately fatal disease for some patients, at the same time larger numbers of cancer patients than ever before can look forward to cure and/or extended survival with their disease as a result of improved cancer treatment. For example, 5-year survival rates over the past several decades have climbed from 4 to 56 percent for acute lymphocytic leukemia, from 63 to 87 percent for testicular cancer, and from 50 to 71 percent for prostate cancer.[5] The intensive cancer treatments that have enabled patients to survive are not without consequences, however, and research is beginning to document persistent and late-emerging effects in survivors.[6,7] Cancer survivors require new approaches to rehabilitation treatment and research, including the development of methods of tracking and monitoring patients over time.

Difficulties in Outcome Assessment

With regard to cancer treatment, the impact of life-saving or life-extending treatments is appropriately measured by relatively unambiguous, easy to assess, and easy to record measures such as mortality and disease-free survival. Such data are routinely maintained on a large scale through cancer registries, which provide an ongoing comprehensive database.

In contrast, the kinds of outcomes appropriate for rehabilitation—improvements in quality of life, enhancement in levels of functioning, and so forth—are difficult to define and even more difficult to measure. The Karnofsky

Performance Index,[8] which was developed to measure functional performance, has been the most widely used instrument to date; however, it can only assess broad levels of performance and cannot indicate differences across levels of functioning. There have been efforts in recent years to develop valid and reliable cancer-specific instruments in areas such as quality of life[9] and rehabilitation problems,[10] and such instruments hold promise for the future. However, many scales that do exist require a great deal of time to administer, record, and analyze, which makes their widespread usage in clinical settings unlikely. Without a widely accepted outcome assessment instrument, it is impossible to generate a database such as a cancer registry, which would greatly facilitate cancer rehabilitation research.

The Multidisciplinary Nature of Cancer Rehabilitation

Many professionals may be involved in delivering rehabilitation: physiatrists, physical therapists, occupational therapists, nurses, social workers, psychologists, and, depending on specific problems, others, such as maxillofacial prosthodontists and speech therapists. In addition, cancer specialists involved in the rehabilitation process, either initially or on an ongoing basis, include medical oncologists, surgeons, and radiation therapists. None of these professions can be said to be the "lead" discipline for cancer rehabilitation therapy or research. Training programs, philosophies of care, vocabularies, priority outcomes, and outlets for publication all vary enormously among rehabilitation professionals. This diversity of expertise poses additional problems for developing and implementing rehabilitation research.

FUTURE DIRECTIONS FOR CANCER REHABILITATION RESEARCH

Progress in cancer rehabilitation research requires attention to issues arising in several phases within the spectrum of cancer control research, from hypothesis development and methodological advances through intervention trials and on to studies that will provide a basis for the dissemination and widespread adoption of rehabilitation practices.[11]

Basic Research

Methodological work is needed on strategies to monitor patients over long periods of time and minimize missing data in longitudinal research. Research is also critically needed to develop outcome assessment instruments that satisfy requirements for validity and reliability and are clinically meaningful and practical to use. The emergence of certain instruments as "standards" in cancer rehabilitation research would facilitate communication among investigators and enhance comparability of findings across multiple settings.

Common instrumentation would also provide a basis for a descriptive epidemiologic database to document the incidence of rehabilitation problems, including treatment morbidity and late effects. If this information could be documented in a form that would allow rehabilitation outcomes to be added to cancer registries, rehabilitation research would have a firm baseline from which to evaluate the impact of future interventions. Especially needed are descriptive studies of rehabilitation problems in populations that are expected to expand in the coming years, such as cancer survivors and the elderly.[12]

Intervention Research

The few available systematic research reports have documented the effectiveness of existing rehabilitation programs, and such studies are sorely needed, as well as trials of innovative approaches. In research design, intervention studies need to incorporate consideration of the heterogeneity of cancer sites, treatments, and patient problems. In order to have sufficient statistical power and to answer research questions more quickly, multicenter trials may be necessary. While clinical cooperative groups, which coordinate trials across multiple centers, have been the primary mechanism for cancer treatment research, little rehabilitation research has been reported by these groups. Utilization of the clinical trial groups for rehabilitation research or development of a new network of researchers for cancer rehabilitation offers the possibility for greatly expanding the scope and generalizability of research in this area.

Dissemination of Research Findings

For rehabilitation interventions to become "standard care," additional research is required. For example, cost-effectiveness is becoming an increasingly important aspect of health care, and any part of the cancer care system must be able to justify its costs in relation to the benefits it provides. Studies of the econometrics of cancer rehabilitation, as well as broad areas of health services research examining the impact of rehabilitation services on the entire system of care, are virtually nonexistent, and yet the need for this kind of information is escalating.

It is clear that research in cancer rehabilitation, like research in therapy, is a multidisciplinary enterprise. Participation by all members of the rehabilitation team throughout the study is critical to maximize chances that the study will be seen as significant and sound in its hypothesis, methodology, and interpretation. Involvement by a broad group is also necessary to ensure that the research will actually be implemented as planned, since most rehabilitation research requires participation by a number of people; referral of all appropriate patients, access to needed information, and data collection and recording as specified in the research protocol are all areas in which commitment by different professionals is needed for the research project to proceed successfully.

Cancer rehabilitation research is an area in which many of the most important questions have not even been asked, let alone answered. Although it is a difficult field in which to conduct research, the potential rewards for the researcher, practitioner, and ultimately for patients and families are considerable.

REFERENCES

1. Ozel AT, Kottke FJ: Research trends in physical medicine and rehabilitation. Arch Phys Med Rehabil 59:166, 1978
2. Gotay CC, Yates JW: Emerging trends in cancer rehabilitation research. p. 18. In Proceedings of the Fifth National Conference on Human Values and Cancer. American Cancer Society, New York, 1987
3. Grabois M, Fuhrer MJ: Physiatrists' views on research. Am J Phys Med Rehabil 67:171, 1988
4. Dietz JH Jr: Rehabilitation Oncology. John Wiley & Sons, Somerset NJ, 1981
5. Page HS, Asire AJ: Cancer Risks and Rates. 3rd Ed. National Cancer Institute, National Institutes of Health, Public Health Service, U.S. Department of Health and Human Services, Washington, 1985
6. Byrd R: Late effects of treatment of cancer in children. Pediatr Clin North Am 32:835, 1985
7. Dobkin PL, Morrow GR: Long-term side effects in patients who have been treated successfully for cancer. J Psychosoc Oncol 3:23, 1986
8. Karnofsky DA, Burchenal JH: The clinical evaluation of chemotherapeutic agents in cancer. p. 191. In Macleod CM (ed): Evaluation of Chemotherapeutic Agents. Columbia University Press, New York, 1949
9. Aaronson NK, Beckmann JH (eds): The Quality of Life of Cancer Patients. Raven Press, New York,1987
10. Schag CC, Heinrich RL, Ganz PA: Cancer inventory of problem situations: An instrument for assessing cancer patients' rehabilitation needs. J Psychosoc Oncol 1:11, 1983
11. Greenwald P, Cullen JW: The new emphasis in cancer control. JNCI 74:543, 1985
12. Gotay CC: New directions in cancer rehabilitation. In Proceedings of the Fifth International Conference on Cancer Nursing, Royal Marsden Hospital, London. (in press)

Index

Page numbers followed by *f* indicate figures; those followed by *t* indicate tables.